P9-CLQ-306

# Counseling in Communication Disorders

## A Wellness Perspective

$\mathcal{O}$n Nov. 18, 1995, Itzhak Perlman, the violinist, came on stage to give a concert at Avery Fisher Hall at Lincoln Center in New York City. If you have ever been to a Perlman concert, you know that getting on stage is no small achievement for him. He was stricken with polio as a child, and so he has braces on both legs and walks with the aid of two crutches. To see him walk across the stage one step at a time, painfully and slowly, is an awesome sight. He walks painfully, yet majestically, until he reaches his chair.

Then he sits down, slowly, puts his crutches on the floor, undoes the clasps on his legs, tucks one foot back and extends the other foot forward. Then he bends down and picks up the violin, puts it under his chin, nods to the conductor and proceeds to play. By now, the audience is used to this ritual. They sit quietly while he makes his way across the stage to his chair. They remain reverently silent while he undoes the clasps on his legs. They wait until he is ready to play.

But this time, something went wrong. Just as he finished the first few bars, one of the strings on his violin broke. You could hear it snap—it went off like gunfire across the room. There was no mistaking what that sound meant. There was no mistaking what he had to do. We figured that he would have to get up, put on the clasps again, pick up the crutches and limp his way off stage—to either find another violin or else find another string for this one. But he didn't. Instead, he waited a moment, closed his eyes and then signaled the conductor to begin again.

The orchestra began, and he played from where he had left off. And he played with such passion and such power and such purity as they had never heard before. Of course, anyone knows that it is impossible to play a symphonic work with just three strings. I know that, and you know that, but that night Itzhak Perlman refused to know that. You could see him modulating, changing, re-composing the piece in his head. At one point, it sounded like he was de-tuning the strings to get new sounds from them that they had never made before.

When he finished, there was an awesome silence in the room. And then people rose and cheered. There was an extraordinary outburst of applause from every corner of the auditorium. We were all on our feet, screaming and cheering, doing everything we could to show how much we appreciated what he had done.

He smiled, wiped the sweat from this brow, raised his bow to quiet us, and then he said—not boastfully, but in a quiet, pensive, reverent tone—"You know, sometimes it is the artist's task to find out how much music you can still make with what you have left."

What a powerful line that is. It has stayed in my mind ever since I heard it. And who knows? Perhaps that is the definition of life—not just for artists but for all of us. Here is a man who has prepared all his life to make music on a violin of four strings, who, all of a sudden, in the middle of a concert, finds himself with only three strings; so he makes music with three strings, and the music he made that night with just three strings was more beautiful, more sacred, more memorable, than any that he had ever made before, when he had four strings. So, perhaps our task in this shaky, fast-changing, bewildering world in which we live is to make music, at first with all that we have, and then, when that is no longer possible, to make music with what we have.

Jack Reimer
*The Houston Chronicle*, 1995

# Counseling in Communication Disorders

## A Wellness Perspective

**Audrey L. Holland, PhD**
Regents' Professor Emerita
University of Arizona
Tucson, Arizona

With a Chapter on End-of-Life Issues by

**Stan Goldberg, PhD**
Professor Emeritus
San Francisco State University
San Francisco California

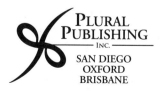

PLURAL
PUBLISHING
INC.

SAN DIEGO
OXFORD
BRISBANE

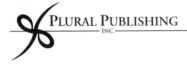

**PLURAL PUBLISHING**
— INC. —

5521 Ruffin Road
San Diego, CA 92123

e-mail: info@pluralpublishing.com
Web site: http://www.pluralpublishing.com

49 Bath Street
Abingdon, Oxfordshire OX14 1EA
United Kingdom

Copyright © by Plural Publishing, Inc. 2007

Typeset in 11/13 Garamond by Flanagan's Publishing Services, Inc.
Printed in the United States of America by Bang Printing

All rights, including that of translation, reserved. No part of this publication
may be reproduced, stored in a retrieval system, or transmitted in any
form or by any means, electronic, mechanical, recording, or otherwise,
including photocopying, recording, taping, Web distribution, or
information storage and retrieval systems without the prior written
consent of the publisher.

For permission to use material from this text, contact us by
Telephone: (866) 758-7251
Fax: (888) 758-7255
e-mail: permissions@pluralpublishing.com

Library of Congress Cataloging-in-Publication Data

Holland, Audrey L.
  Counseling in communication disorders : a wellness perspective /
Audrey L. Holland.
       p. ; cm.
  Includes bibliographical references and index.
  ISBN-13: 978-1-59756-049-8 (pbk.)
  ISBN-10: 1-59756-049-9 (pbk.)
  1. Communicative disorders—Patients—Counseling of. 2. Rehabilitation
counseling. 3. Speech therapy. 4. Audiology. I. Title.
  [DNLM: 1. Communication Disorders. 2. Counseling—methods.
WL 340.2 H734c 2007]
  RC428.8.H6673 2007
  616.85'506—dc22

                                                        2006102015

# CONTENTS

# FOREWORD

"No pessimist ever discovered the secret of the
stars or sailed an uncharted land, or opened a new
doorway for the human spirit."

Helen Keller, U.S. blind and
deaf educator (1880–1968)

This is a book about opening new doorways for people with communication disorders and their families. It is not a "fix-it" book or an intervention book aimed at ferreting out problem behaviors and changing them. As Holland states in Chapter 1, it is a book aimed at emphasizing what is right with people with communication disorders as a means of helping them and their families "mobilize their strengths to deal with the adversities that have befallen them as the result of an unexpected and unplanned for event." By making positive psychology the "theoretical heart" of this book, Holland shows clinicians (whether in training or already experienced) how to help clients and families see their glass not only half-full rather than half-empty, but also to help them fill it even further by identifying and mobilizing their strengths.

This is not the first time I have been impressed by the wisdom of Audrey Holland and her ability to trigger insights in others. Although I have enjoyed and benefited from Holland's work over the years, I have an episodic memory of the first time I encountered it. I was a beginning clinician and reading voraciously anything that might guide me toward "knowing what to do" when facing a child with a language disorder in my clinic room. It was a time when behaviorism was the dominant theory of treatment and when Chomsky's was the dominant voice in explaining language acquisition. It was a fascinating time because controversies were flying; conference presentations often turned into heated debates fueled by passionate claims for firmly staked positions about nature versus nurture. Such arguments were far from abstract for a young clinician drawn to linguistic theoretical explanations but wanting her life's work to involve nurturing change when nature took a wrong turn.

It should have been easy, as only one of the two contrasting positions offered concrete advice about "what to do" to teach language. When I tried the behaviorist approaches of the day; however, I found that they stripped far too much meaning from the forms targeted in intervention. Moreover, I felt that I was triggering communication frustration rather than communication when requiring young children to comply with repetitive massed trials, such as endless requests to "Stand up" then "Sit down," or to imitate as in, "The girl is eating, Alison, say is," to earn token or food reinforcers. Nor did such approaches allow any appreciation of, or intervention for, the social-emotional aspects of communication difficulties. On the other hand, linguistic theorists discouraged the concept that language was even teachable. What was one to do?

The possibilities of another approach based on social-interaction and contextualizing the need for language forms first dawned for me in an "aha" moment while reading an article written by Audrey Holland (1975) in the *Journal of Speech and Hearing Disorders* (which later became subsumed under the *Journal of Speech, Language, and Hearing Research*). Bloom (1970) had published her monograph on *Language development: Form and function of emerging grammars*, but Bates (1976) had yet to publish *Language and context: The acquisition of pragmatics*. Regardless, it was Holland's article that made social-interactionist theory come alive for me as the means to making communication intervention both meaningful and joyful. The essence was the story of a clinical session with a young child struggling with early language, which entailed pulling tissues from a box and tossing them in the air while shouting "More!" That story painted a new picture for me. I was hooked. This was the kind of clinician I wanted to be. Holland helped me see that the key was to be found in understanding the social contexts of communication interactions and my job was to help create them. Within such meaningful social contexts, I could provide the mediating supports so that my clients could be more successful than they could be on their own.

In this book, more stories of the possibilities of change and "aha" moments are to be found as Holland applies her views of social-interactionism, contextualizing, and mediating communicative experiences to the realm of communication counseling. Holland's focus on wellness and making use of everyday experiences helps to establish clarity for the counseling roles speech-language pathologists and audiologists can and should play with their clients, while establishing boundaries against assuming roles that should be played by other professionals, who are fully prepared to address psychopathology. At the same time, Holland does not minimize the significance of the "catastrophic" feelings associated the "wrenching problems" of communication disorders across the lifespan; nor does she deny their impact on multiple aspects of life. What she does is illuminate the role of clinicians in helping clients find the positive elements of life with the disorder, beyond the disorder, and aside from the disorder.

As a person whose work centers on the needs of children and adolescents and their families, I was particularly drawn to Holland's chapters on counseling children and their parents. Critical distinctions are associated with different points of parental awareness. In Chapter 4, Holland focuses on how communication counseling should proceed when the bad news comes early, even in the prenatal stages of a child's development. In her straightforward way, Holland helps her readers look out through the eyes of parents of newborns, when the parents suddenly must cope with the realization that their idealized perfect child has Down syndrome or a craniofacial anomaly. In Chapter 5, Holland guides readers to switch perspective to that of parents who first experience a period of development with their child when all appears well, only to discover later that their child's communication abilities are affected by stuttering, specific language impairment, or other late-appearing syndromes. For such parents, either hearing the news from others, or gaining gradual awareness themselves leads to internal conflict with what Holland calls the parents' views on "the child who used to be." Also in Chapter 5, Holland addresses the needs of parents whose children acquire their difficulties suddenly through traumatic events, such as vehicular accidents.

Perhaps the most paradigm nudging concept that Holland includes in this book is to distinguish this form of communication counseling from others required for dealing with forms psychopathology. As Holland points out in Chapter 1, most people who can benefit from communication counseling are "likely to have been coping with their lives fairly normally before the onset of the communication disorder." Like many elegantly simple concepts, this one seems obvious once encountered.

Other favorite elements of the book for me are Holland's characterization of the role of communication counseling as being one of coaching and her emphasis on the value of stories. In the case of coaching, she notes that speech-language pathologists and audiologists can capitalize on their knowledge of how to teach people to change their communication skills and can apply it to learning related roles for coaching clients and families to be resilient and optimistic in facing life's challenges.

In the case of Holland's emphasis on the use of stories, I was stimulated to reconsider some old writings by Jerome Bruner (1986) and to seek out some of his newer work (Bruner, 2004) on the multi-level meaning of narratives. As I read the many stories Holland has included in this book, I was struck again by the power of narratives to help people come to grips with life events over which they may have little control. Using the concepts of dual narrative landscapes that Bruner (1986, 2004) popularized (citing Greimus & Courtes, 1976), the essence of helping people construct new possibilities for themselves can be found in helping them distinguish the landscape of consciousness from the *landscape of action*. Within the landscape of consciousness, characters exert choices for regrouping, responding, and proceeding when catastrophic events befall them; without such consciousness, all that is left is an essentially passive landscape of action, in which things *happen to* the main characters, but over which they exert little thought or control. Bruner (2004) expanded on the power of culturally shaped cognitive and linguistic processes for guiding the self-telling of life narratives. He noted that such process can "achieve the power to structure perceptual experience, to organize memory, to segment and purpose-build the very 'events' of a life" (p. 196). Bruner concluded:

> My life as a student of mind has taught me one incontrovertible lesson: mind is never free of precommitment. There is no innocent eye, nor is there one that penetrates aboriginal reality. There are instead hypotheses, versions, expected scenarios. Our precommitment about the nature of a life is that it is a story, some narrative however incoherently put together. Perhaps we can say one other thing: any story one may tell about anything is better understood by considering other possible ways in which it can be told. (p. 709)

Holland's gift is her ability to help others envision multiple possibilities for telling their stories. It is a gift I came to value early in my career and appreciate even more now. This book shows clinicians how to open new doorways to the resilience of the human spirit and how to help clients and families construct their lives—both beyond communication disorders and with them.

Nickola Wolf Nelson, PhD
Charles Van Riper Professor
Department of Speech Pathology and Audiology
Western Michigan University, Kalamazoo

## References

Bates, E. (1976). *Language and context: The acquisition of pragmatics.* New York: Academic Press.

Bloom, L. (1970). *Language development: Form and function of emerging grammars.* Research Monograph No. 59. Cambridge, MA: The M.I.T. Press.

Bruner, J. (1986). *Actual minds, possible worlds.* Cambridge: Harvard University Press.

Bruner, J. (2004). Life as narrative. *Social Research: An International Quarterly of Social Sciences, 71*(3), 691–710.

Greimas, A., & Courtes, J. (Spring 1976). The cognitive dimension of narrative discourse. *New Literary History, 7.* (cited by Bruner, 2004)

Holland, A. (1975). Language therapy for children: Some thoughts on context and content. *Journal of Speech and Hearing Disorders, 40,* 514–523.

Keller, H. Quotation retrieved on 12/26/06 from http://www.quotationspage.com/quote/32595.html

# PREFACE

$\mathcal{T}$his book comes from my heart. It is not meant to be a scientific treatise on counseling; rather, it describes a counseling *attitude*, and explores how speech language pathologists can enrich clinical practice using specific skills and techniques incorporating that attitude. It also embodies a set of principles that began as ruminations on professional observations, developed over my many years of clinical work as an SLP and in formal clinical research. For some years I contemplated writing a book about the softer side of the profession: its counseling agenda. For most of my career, I have tried to keep my scientific practice in step with my humanistic practice because I believe truly productive clinical work results from their judicious blending. So that is what this book is about.

Practitioners and students who are interested only in the particulars of clients who might comprise the bulk of their caseloads should be aware that there are no shortcuts in this book. I have emphasized a "lifespan perspective," requiring an appreciation of the backward and forward interplay between the different life phases: Down syndrome toddlers grow older, dementia happens to people who have previously led smooth and mostly uneventful lives, but who may profit from what people with lifelong problems may have to offer. Sadly, death happens across the lifespan.

Counseling (or Coaching as I prefer to call it, although the less formal, more active connotation has not yet been accepted across our disciplines), as it is instantiated here, requires holistic understanding. The result is that all of this book's chapters relate to each other. Thus, reading this book requires some attention to all of it, rather than seeking out bits and pieces of it to study more intensively. That doesn't mean that you can toss it across the room at the end of one of the chapters and never look at it again! It just means that there is an inevitable intertwining, and that to get the most out of the book, you have to "go the distance."

I have loved writing this book—the nature of work of the heart, I suspect. I have especially loved the notion of awakening some readers to the potential of positive psychology, not only for clients but also for themselves. I have cherished the interactions with others involved in the creation of this text and the feedback I have received. Please enjoy reading it—I hope it is a meaningful experience for you.

Namasté

# ACKNOWLEDGMENTS

The people who helped with preparation of this book are too numerous to acknowledge here, and of those who are named, it's almost impossible to determine whose contribution was in fact greatest. This inability to decide on an appropriate order of the many recipients of my gratitude is especially significant to me because the quality of "gratitude" was painfully, embarrassingly, in middle territory on the Values in Action (VIA) assessment an inventory of character strengths and virtues central to Positive Psychology. I took this inventory a few years ago.and since then, I have been working to improve my ability to express gratitude, and I don't want to miss a single person.

So I'm just going to do this willy-nilly, beginning with the Ongoing Pod, my inspirational phone-in group of weekly discussants and celebrants. We have been meeting since the spring of 2004, and few of us have actually seen each other, but we surely do connect nonetheless. Pod members are Brian Branigan, Linda Emerson, Gerissa French, Bill Hefferman, Frank Mosca, and (sometimes showing up, but always there in spirit) David Pollay. Karen Reivich, who wins "the most-frequently quoted" award for this book, has been Pod leader from the beginning, and all I want to say about Karen is that I would be proud to be her mother, in addition to being Ben and Kate's. You all have been there for me, and I cannot thank you enough, especially—the whole Pod would agree—Karen.

Then there are the people who helped me with the material on children: Noel Matkin, who put in time and provided sage advice on Chapters 4 and 5; Tony DeFeo, a fantastic critic and clinician who gave me hope that these ideas were not crazy: Patrick Finn and Nan Ratner, who taught me about stuttering; Alice Smith, Trudi Murch, and Jeanne Wilcox, who listened and responded to my worries about kids and the spectrum of their disabilities; Cynthia Kidder and Sue Swenson, who shaped my parent perspectives; and Katie Holland, who added another parent perspective, but who also cleared up my pediatric medical errors, and listened to me, her mother, in incredibly helpful ways.

Also of invaluable help were the many adult-focused experts, who were both positive and informative. Cindy Thompson, in fact, got me into this in the first place, largely as a result of her listening to me and poking and prodding me to go with it. I am also grateful for the listening and prodding of many others. Here they are, in no specific order whatsoever: Lyn Turkstra, Nina Simmons-Mackie, Ursula Bellugi, Jan Avent, Leslie Gonzalez Rothi, Aura Kagan, Edie Strand, Roberta Elman, the Michaels Chial and Flahive, Anita Halper, Leora Cherney—and Stan Goldberg, in a place by himself.

There is also a special list of people who worked with my conceptualizations, my writing prolixities, and my lapses in logic and sensibility: the Singhs, first of all, but also Adina Newberg, Margie Forbes, Jane Dominick, Fabi Hirsch, Tina Bronson-Lowe, Joan Eisenberg, and Cathy Fay—this book would still be in working manuscript" form without you. And thanks to Louise Serpa, who generously gave me permission to use one of her photographs for the cover of this book

A special acknowledgment belongs to the participants in my HIV-AIDS workshop in the summer of 2005, where I worked through many of these ideas. You lovely people know who you are, and also that you truly challenged, delighted, and taught me. Thank you.

And thanks as well to my 2005 counseling class, who "test drove" many of these then half-formed ideas and patiently evaluated them. I don't know how much counseling you learned that term, but you saved many current readers from some of my rather stunning disasters, and you certainly taught me a lot.

Thanks greatly to Martin E. P. Seligman for the beautiful long-distance master class in positive psychology he taught to 400 eager learners around the world in the spring of 2004. The course was one of the most eye-popping experiences of my life, and, I hope, clear proof that old dogs *can* learn new tricks.

Finally, know that this is not the first book on counseling that has ever been written in our field. It might seem that I have paid scant attention to those whose work preceded me. I have not avoided them, but because this book takes a somewhat different perspective, I chose not to get sidetracked into what we share and don't share and where we agree or disagree. But my respect for these scholars is boundless, and I owe them much. These people include Lydia Flasher, Paul Fogle , David Luterman, Walter Rollin and George Shames. I am aware that I am riding, perhaps pretty insecurely, on a lot of very big shoulders.

To Betty Webster and Louise Ward, for their inestimable influence on me, and others whose lives they touched so deeply.

To Ben and Katie, who both continue to teach me, in different ways, about different things, but what would I have become without you? I love you.

And to my beloved grandchildren, Adrian, Thomas, and Anne.

*Chapter 1*

# COUNSELING IN CLINICAL PRACTICE: OVERVIEW

*S*peech-language pathologists and audiologists (SLP-As) bring expertise in specific clinical areas to the evaluation and management of communication disorders. Additionally, an important skill for both students and practicing clinicians to develop is effective counseling of clients and their families to support decisions and behaviors that optimize quality of life. Knowledge of effective counseling techniques supplements the professional's knowledge about communication disorders and his or her skills in managing these disorders. Appropriate counseling greatly increases the opportunity for an optimal outcome for clients, whether this involves resolving a specific disorder or maximizing quality of life by means of coping and adjustment techniques.

With many communication disorders, the role of the speech-language-hearing professionals is complex. Children with severe hearing losses or cerebral palsy and their families, for example, face lifelong struggles. Complex problems arise at the other end of the age spectrum as well: Adults who acquire aphasia, for example, must learn to deal with profoundly changed lives. The clinical goal for individuals with communication disorders is certainly to minimize the disorder's effects, but counseling also can help involved persons to live productively and successfully with the communication problems, or despite them, or around them.

1

According to the American Speech-Language-Hearing Association's (ASHA) Scope of Practice statements for speech-language pathology (2001) and for audiology (2004), counseling is an integral part of clinical responsibility for families and children with speech, language, and hearing disorders, as well as for adults who have acquired such disorders. Counseling is perhaps the most important way we SLP-As have to help our clients achieve lifelong goals. SLP-As often feel uncomfortable about the counseling role, however, and consequently tend to avoid it.

A number of reasons may underlie this reluctance. Perhaps a lack of explicit training in counseling explains it. During our professional education, we are given a wealth of information about the potential problems confronting individuals and families with communication disorders but are taught very little about how the counseling process can be used to help resolve them. Indeed, the ASHA provides no curriculum requirements for counseling. If counseling is presented at all in SLP-A training, it is likely to be tagged onto the end of disorder-specific courses, rather than presented in its own right as a skill to be learned through coursework and practice.

General counseling principles and skills can be fitted to specific problems. The techniques and skills are similar for helping a family with a new baby who has a cleft palate or a hearing deficit and for supporting an adult client with post-stroke aphasia and his family, who face the realities of living with impaired communication. Only the disorder-specific facts differ.

I suspect that another factor contributing to the reluctance of SLP-As to assume a counseling role is the often negative connotation of "counseling" in the context of psychopathology. A majority of the counseling approaches used with individuals who have communication disorders were borrowed from a perspective in clinical psychology that stresses the detrimental behavioral effects of some types of psychopathology, principally disorders that occur along the depression continuum. For example, counseling individuals who stutter traditionally has been heavily influenced by nondirective approaches, as exemplified by Carl Rogers' client-centered therapy (1995). Similarly, although Freudian defense mechanisms may have interesting implications for anxiety disorders, they offer little for a family whose financial anxieties stem from the breadwinner's Parkinson's disease or incapacitation following a motor vehicle accident.

People who are in need of communication counseling are likely to have been coping with their lives fairly normally before the onset of the communication disorder. This is not to say that individuals with psychological or behavioral problems are immune to communication problems, but a majority of the people for whom SLP-As provide counseling or coaching probably react to the world in ways that are not pathological. The abnormal models of counseling do not fit very well; accordingly, they are difficult to apply in clinical practice, even if we have taken a course or two in abnormal psychology. Most communication problems have unique, significant, and reverberating effects on families, who are likely to be as unprepared for them as those who actually incur the problems. Our discipline's reliance on abnormal psychology has seldom been questioned or examined, although it may explain at least partially why many practitioners feel uneasy with their counseling roles.

In this book, counseling for communication disorders has a different theoretical perspective. This approach requires essentially abandoning a treatment model based on what is *wrong* with people who have such disorders. Instead, the emphasis is on what is *right* with them, and how they can mobilize their strengths to deal with the adversities that have befallen them as the result of an unexpected and unplanned-for event that threatens one of the most basic human characteristics—the ability to communicate. Thus, the counseling process starts with the assumption that the cup is half full, not half empty. Before onset or recognition of a communication disorder, the affected person—whether an adult client who has experienced a stroke with resultant aphasia or the parent of a newborn infant who has been found to be at risk for such a disorder, for example—probably already has been coping reasonably well with life stresses. How do we as counselors capitalize on and build on the positive?

## Themes of Interest

Five themes that focus on how to help individuals with communication disorders to develop optimism and resilience constitute a framework for this book. These themes are described next, in no implied hierarchy; all are equally important.

## Theme 1: Wellness and Positive Psychology

Much of the content of this book is based on a conviction that appropriate models and approaches for communication counseling should be grounded in what we know about normality and wellness, rather than in what we know about illness and psychopathology. The recent explosion of information about and interest in positive psychology provides the best example, particularly as it is illuminated by the work of Seligman and his colleagues (e.g., Haidt, 2006; Peterson, 2006; Reivich & Shatté, 2002; Seligman, 1991, 2002; Snyder & Lopez, 2005).

Thus, the first theme of this book is its reliance on the principles and tenets of *positive psychology*, focusing on mental health and well-being and how to achieve and maintain them. Positive psychology is oriented away from illness and toward wellness, both for understanding what it means to live positively and for providing ways to increase authentic happiness in one's own life. This book links those principles to counseling individuals and families who experience and live with communication disorders.

One of the most appealing aspects of focusing on wellness and positive psychology as a counseling model in communication disorders is that it fits squarely with the facet of counseling with which SLP-As are most comfortable: providing information. We are skilled educators and good providers of information. Training in speech-language pathology and audiology produces good teachers— whether we are teaching children to move a lateral lisp into a more acceptable /s/ production, or reestablishing semantic skills in aphasic adults, or teaching effective hearing aid use. Counseling is a change process, as are many of the other techniques used by SLP-As. To the extent that our counseling can capitalize on our teaching skills, we can become comfortable with a counseling role.

A core feature of positive psychology is its development of explicit ways to increase resilience and optimism. These two attributes are particularly critical for learning to cope with the many disasters or catastrophes that occur in the process of simply living life. Basic principles of positive psychology are covered in Chapter 2, and a number of its experimentally validated exercises are presented there. Other exercises that have been adapted specifically for communication counseling are scattered throughout the book.

## Theme 2:  Living the Catastrophe

In this book, the words *catastrophe* and *catastrophic* generally are used in the conventional sense of *disaster* and *disastrous*. They imply the kinds of wrenching problems that result from the spectrum of communication disorders ranging from developmental disorders discovered in infancy to the dementias that occur late in life. But *catastrophe* also is used in this book in the sense that Jon Kabat-Zinn used it in his book on stress reduction and meditation, *Full Catastrophe Living* (anniversary edition, 2005). Kabat-Zinn borrowed his title in part from Kazantzakis' *Zorba the Greek* (1996). In the film adaptation of Kazantzakis' book, Zorba responds to the question of whether he was ever married: "Of course I've been married. Wife, house, kids, everything . . . the full catastrophe!" Kabat-Zinn interpreted Zorba's remark as a basic appreciation of the roller-coaster nature of being alive. This usage of the word *catastrophe* embodies the spirit of accepting change and knowing that, in Kabat-Zinn's words,

> . . . it is not a disaster to be alive just because we feel fear and we suffer . . . [to understand] that there is joy as well as suffering, hope as well as despair, calm as well as agitation, love as well as hatred, health as well as illness . . . (p. 5)

The "full catastrophe" for most people involves good *and* bad, easy *and* hard, periods of happiness *and* periods of pain. In fact, someone who manages to avoid the negatives may be perceived in some way as diminished (and perhaps likely to be rather boring!). Although the issues we deal with in our communication counseling gravitate toward the negative pole, it is crucial to remember that the opposite, the positive, also is there. Good counselors respect and honor not only their clients and their problems but also the "full catastrophe" of the human condition.

## Theme 3:  Who Are the Experts?

The social model of disability, which has been growing in strength and influence over the past 30 years has significant implications for the practice of speech-language pathology and audiology in general. Perhaps its greatest significance relates to our professions' counseling functions. Briefly put, the social model makes it clear that disability itself is hardly a problem of disabled persons alone; it also is a substantial result of living in disabling societies. Furthermore, disability is perhaps not a tragedy but a fact of life (part of the whole catastrophe, as it were). Finally, the problems faced by people with disabilities are broad social ones, requiring similarly broad social solutions and sweeping attitudinal change on the part of the nondisabled, including the professionals who work with them.

The disability movement (Barnes, Mercer, & Shakespeare, 1999; Oliver, 1996) embodies those social concerns and has had a significant impact on the development of the International Classification of Functioning and Disability (ICF) (World Health Organization, 2001). Although full discussion of the ICF is beyond the scope of this book, it is a topic with which all SLP-As must become familiar. One important implication for counseling is that the social model of disability insists that societies rethink the question of expertise in relation to any disabling condition. It asks the question "Who is the expert?" This question has powerful ramifications for counseling. People with disabilities have strongly challenged the traditional assumption that *professional* is synonymous with *expert*. In this book, that challenge is endorsed by acknowledgment of the expertise of clients and families.

The initial approach to counseling should recognize that as SLP-As, we have an undeniable expertise consisting of our technical knowledge and our ability to compile the resources that might be available to our clients. But does this expertise ensure that we are *the* experts? In fact, at least one and possibly two or three other experts are involved. One expert is the person who lives *in* the disorder. (This is particularly relevant for adolescents and adults who live with communication disorders) The other experts are those who live *with* the disorder. This means families and significant others. In much the same way in which meaning in conversation is co-constructed by a speaker and a listener, counseling is co-constructed by these experts—that is, the disabled person, those whose lives are connected to the disabled person, and the counselor.

This expanded concept of "expert" became clear to me even before the advent of the social model of disability. As a beginning clinician, I often found myself smugly amused when parents would comment about their child, "He never acts like this at home." "Hmm," I would think—"it's amazing what sort of blinders parents wear, particularly if experts aren't around." And then I had children. The first time I heard myself utter, "He isn't like this at home," I recognized my limitations as an expert. I learned that as clinicians, we could claim only one of the two or three places at the experts' table.

## Theme 4: The Importance of Stories

The fourth theme of this book involves narrative as it relates to problem solving and counseling. Telling one's own story as part of the healing process that precedes the development of resilience and optimism is crucial. Such narratives contain a lot of the narrator's power; see the writings of Coles (1989), Frank (1995), and Kleinman (1988) for excellent examples of the genre of illness narrative. Hinckley (2006) has recently addressed this topic in relation to stories written by persons with aphasia and their families.

In his novel *Still Life with Woodpecker* (1980), Tom Robbins notes that we "all star in our own movie." This is a profound notion.[1] We learn from ourselves as we hear ourselves tell our own stories. We also learn when we listen to each other's stories (in effect, when we "see" each other's movies), and derive important lessons and role models from them. A sage aphasic client pointed out that one of the most healing aspects of his aphasia group was the frequent ritual of each group member telling the story of his or her stroke and the progress away from it. These stories never lost their centrality, and each new member was always welcomed into the group with telling and sharing the stories of the veteran group members, as well as the story of the new member.

Accordingly, stories about real people with real communication problems appear frequently throughout this book. These stories are positive, but usually not heroic. They are simply everyday instances of getting along with life, of moving on. They reflect the importance of positive attitudes and behaviors, and they serve to remind us of the importance of finding and using such stories and role models in counseling.

---

[1]But Pema Chodron (2001) counters with the following: "It is possible to move through the drama of our lives without believing so earnestly in the character we play." This serves as a reminder of our role in the big scheme of things, and of our need for perspective.

## Theme 5: Crisis

The final theme of this book is understanding and using a crisis model in communication counseling. First developed by Elisabeth Kübler-Ross for dealing with grief, death, and dying (1969), a crisis model has been useful with many chronic health issues as well. Although it has significant shortcomings, this model, as adapted by Webster and Newhoff (1981) for our professions, can be useful for elucidating the process whereby individuals can learn to deal with catastrophic events. Webster and Newhoff discuss the relevance of a crisis approach for counseling families and individuals after stroke. The model has been widely adapted for a spectrum of disorders and conditions.

Specifically, four stages are postulated to occur as individuals progress toward healthy resolution. These stages are called various names by various authors. In this book, Webster and Newhoff's terms are used. These are, in order, *shock*, *realization*, *retreat*, and *acknowledgment*. Certainly, not all individuals go through all stages in an orderly fashion, and not all individuals actually reach satisfactory acknowledgment. In fact, Goldberg (2006) recently commented that in his extensive experience as a hospice counselor, he has never observed an individual who followed precisely these stages of grief. Nevertheless, these stages provide a model that is important for SLP-As to keep in mind as they conduct counseling related to communication (as supported by clinical experience with counseling clients with aphasia at the University of Arizona Aphasia Clinic).

Immediately after an aphasia-producing stroke, neither the family nor the person who has experienced it is in a particularly good position to take advantage of information concerning stroke-related aphasia offered at that time. Nevertheless, almost without exception, experienced clinicians routinely provide such information. Frequently, however, SLP-As whose work focuses on chronic aphasia hear comments from clients and their families that "things were not explained" and that they had no idea what to expect. In such instances, the shock of the stroke may compromise the ability of both the affected person and family members to absorb new information in the earliest stages of recovery. This limitation does not mean that clinicians should stop providing information in the initial aftermath of a potentially disabling event. But we should not be surprised when affected individuals and families fail to comprehend all of the early information they receive, and we should be prepared to repeat it, perhaps frequently.

Of greater importance, this initial failure to comprehend or retain relevant information means that the first of Webster's (1977) counseling functions—listening—should be primary. Webster points out that listening to what people wish to share and to their fears about the future, and simply holding hands and being present are what matters at this time. It also is valuable to provide information that is more permanent than the spoken word. Pamphlets, videotapes, and contact information sheets and the like will be useful later, when the realization stage is reached. Once the client and family members realize what this problem may actually entail, written information and relevant phone numbers can be used productively.

Retreat is likely to be the least universal of these four crisis stages, at least for the types of problems encountered by SLP-As. However, retreat can manifest itself in denial that a problem actually exists or that the disorder will have a major impact in the long run. For example, Dora, the spouse of a man who has recently suffered a stroke, comments, "Ralph may have global aphasia, but you don't know his will. He'll be back to work at his old job in 6 months, mark my words." As counselors, we must be aware of the delicate nature of such denial, as well as of the need to deal with denial when it occurs.

It is common in the Aphasia Clinic at the University of Arizona Clinic for families of aphasic individuals who have been recently discharged from rehabilitation centers to provide ratings of their spouse's communication ability using the Communication Effectiveness Index (CETI) (Lomas et al., 1989) that are substantially higher than CETI scores obtained six months later. After families have lived with a disorder for a longer period of time, problems often become more apparent. When Dora realizes Ralph is not back at work yet, and that their future may be very different from the one she has envisioned, counseling offers the mechanism for her reassessment.

Acknowledgment of the problem is not a synonym for *giving up*. It is recognizing the reality of the individual's condition, making room for the changes, and moving on with life. Ram Dass, who completed his book *Still Here* (2001) after experiencing a stroke that resulted in aphasia and hemiplegia, eloquently described the good that resulted from acknowledging his deficit. He comments:

> The stroke was like a samurai sword, cutting apart the two halves of my life. It was a demarcation between the two stages. In a way, it's been like having two incarnations in one; this is me that was "him" . . . Seeing it that way saves me from the suffering of making comparisons, of thinking about the things I used to do but can't do any more because of the paralysis in my hand. In the "past incarnation" I had an MG with a stick shift, I had golf clubs, I had a cello. Now I don't have any use for those things! New incarnation! (Ram Dass, 2000)

Wellness and positive psychology, the full catastrophe, shared expertise, illness narrative, and crisis are essential elements of the counseling approach developed in this book. These elements form the basis for the concepts, techniques, skills, and exercises presented throughout the text as tools to increase the effectiveness of SLP-As in counseling clients and families across the spectrum of communication disorders. First, however, a number of definitions need to be clarified to permit their use as a kind of shorthand in the rest of this book. Finally, a few other topics such as the role of group and individual counseling are dealt with briefly in this overview.

## Definitions

Box 1.1 presents the components of counseling in communication disorders. The first step in learning the counseling process is to define it, and to set the boundaries around counseling in speech-language pathology and audiology.

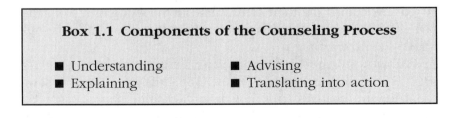

**Box 1.1 Components of the Counseling Process**

- Understanding
- Explaining
- Advising
- Translating into action

## What Is Counseling in Communication Disorders?

Counseling is, above all, a listening process. The first task of this listening process involves trying to understand how the world looks to the client. This requires careful self-examination of the SLP-A's personal, subjective worldview, and then systematically taking the steps necessary to remove personal biases that would compromise the listening process. Once unbiased listening has been learned and practiced, we can apply it in our counseling for clients whose worldview, cultural beliefs, and personal principles may differ significantly from our own. The ability to see how the world looks to our clients provides the context of understanding and acceptance that makes them comfortable enough to express their feelings, concerns, anxieties, and so forth. The second task of counseling is to encourage such expression. The clinical atmosphere for counseling must be such that a client feels safe, as well as cherished and respected. The third task in the counseling process is advising— that is, providing the information that people need to help them understand what is happening to them, as well as showing them how to get on with their lives and live in a realistic fashion, with both optimism and resilience. Then comes the last task of counseling and the most difficult step: helping individuals to translate information into satisfying and successful actions.

The goal of the counseling process is to help individuals and families to live as successfully as they possibly can, despite the intrusion of such events as a motor vehicle accident that results in a child's traumatic brain injury, a stroke that occurs just as retirement is nearing, a dawning awareness of an infant's developmental disability, or any of a score of other catastrophic events that result in communication disorders.

The major aspects of communication counseling were identified some years ago by Webster (1977), as follows:

- To receive information that the individual and his or her family wish to share with you
- To give information
- To help individuals clarify their ideas, attitudes, emotions, and beliefs
- To provide options for changing behaviors

Note that this last point does *not* mean prescribing therapy or even necessarily advocating for a particular form of intervention. It merely means providing all of the information necessary for clients to make their own informed decisions from among the range of alternatives.

The intent of counseling with communicatively impaired persons and their families is to help them achieve the following:

- To grieve what has been lost
- To understand what has happened as fully as possible
- To develop coping strategies and to increase resilience
- To make peace with the disorder
- To make sensible adaptations to the disorder
- To capitalize on strengths in order to minimize weaknesses
- To live as fully as possible, despite impairment

## What Is *Not* Counseling in Communication Disorders?

Although frequently taught together, counseling and interviewing have different goals and are merely related processes. A veritable chasm separates taking a case history from listening to a story and reacting appropriately to that story. *Interviewing* is the skill of finding out about another (in this case, someone with a communication disorder or a family member) through perceptive questioning and observation. In contrast with the counseling goals described earlier, the goal of interviewing is to provide the clinician with valid and pertinent information that informs the entire clinical process, including appropriate methods of intervention. This book is not about interviewing—it is about communication counseling.

Because the primary training of SLP-As is in communication sciences and disorders, not in clinical psychology or psychiatry, our clinical skills have implicit boundaries. Practically every specialized counseling textbook stresses the importance of placing some limits to counseling performed by the respective specialists. Counseling in our disciplines is no exception. The ASHA Scope of Practice statements for both audiology and speech-language pathology (ASHA, 2001, 2004) limit our counseling responsibilities to those that relate to communication disorders.

As counselors to clients with communication disorders, we are not clinical psychologists, and as is reiterated throughout this book, one of our primary sensitivities must be to know when our skills are not enough, and when referrals to other professionals such as psychiatrists, psychologists, genetic counselors, or social workers are appropriate. Box 1.2 lists some activities that can be considered outside the scope of practice for communication counselors.

In the remainder of this book, the term *communication counseling* replaces the rather burdensome phrase "counseling individuals and their families who have communication disorders." Use of this term provides a continual reminder of the boundaries of our counseling work.

## Coaching

*Coaching* is a fast-growing new entry in the broad field of the helping professions and is relevant to communication counseling. Thus,

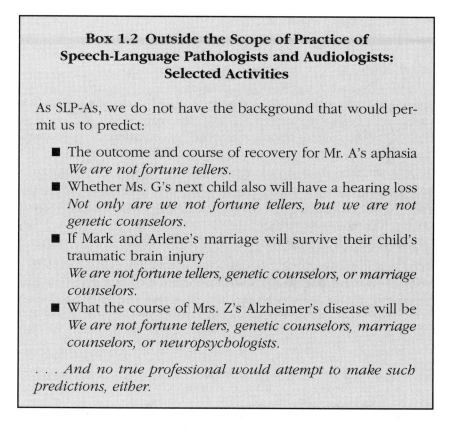

**Box 1.2 Outside the Scope of Practice of Speech-Language Pathologists and Audiologists: Selected Activities**

As SLP-As, we do not have the background that would permit us to predict:

- The outcome and course of recovery for Mr. A's aphasia
  *We are not fortune tellers.*
- Whether Ms. G's next child also will have a hearing loss
  *Not only are we not fortune tellers, but we are not genetic counselors.*
- If Mark and Arlene's marriage will survive their child's traumatic brain injury
  *We are not fortune tellers, genetic counselors, or marriage counselors.*
- What the course of Mrs. Z's Alzheimer's disease will be
  *We are not fortune tellers, genetic counselors, marriage counselors, or neuropsychologists.*

*. . . And no true professional would attempt to make such predictions, either.*

a brief note on coaching is in order here. I am trained as a life coach and practice many of its principles and tactics primarily in helping people (with and without language disorders) to age successfully, and in helping adult children to plan with and support their aging parents. The principles and skills of life coaching provide at least as pertinent a model for SLP-As as that on which more conventionally defined counseling is based. Coaching is a process that is grounded in wellness. Its emphasis is on normalcy and health, on correctly identifying sources of problems and teaching problem-solving skills to apply to them, and developing and implementing pertinent action plans. Coaching also focuses on differentiating those problems that are within a person's ability to control from those that are beyond such control.

## Process-Specific Definitions

### Who Practices Communication Counseling?

Who are the health-related professionals who practice communication counseling? The answer, of course, is SLP-As.

### With Whom Is Communication Counseling Practiced?

In identifying those persons with whom communication counseling is practiced, no term is entirely suitable. The word *patient* implies sickness. The phrase "individuals with speech, language, or hearing disorders" (much less "and their families") seems just to big a mouthful. So for simplicity, currency, and clarity, the term *client* is used throughout this book. Thus, SLP-As practice communication counseling with their clients.[2]

### When Does an SLP-A Provide Counseling?

Communication counselors at times may set aside sessions for counseling their clients. An example of such sessions is the resilience

---

[2]In this context, it is striking how overwrought the language of this discipline is. This is rather ironic, because a basic belief of the professions concerns clear, concise, intelligible, and, for some people, even "functional" language.

and optimism-building workshop models described in Chapter 8. The counseling provided by SLP-As, however, is more likely to be accomplished "on the fly" during more communication-focused intervention sessions with adult clients, for example, when an aphasic man with inconsistent family support may express doubts about the value of this therapy for him, or when a dysarthric woman whose progress has failed to meet her expectations voices her disappointment.

These instances may reveal important relevant information— for example, that sleeping problems are interfering with concentration. Counseling also often gets tucked into brief parent or family encounters at the beginning of a session, before more structured treatment begins, or at its end, when we may be summarizing what happened during the session itself. A useful term for such mini-encounters is "counseling moments"; examples are provided throughout this book. As effective communication counselors, we must be alert for these moments and be prepared to practice our counseling skills in ongoing, small, and even casual interactions throughout more focused clinical interventions.

## A Note on Depression and Communication Sciences

It is necessary to be emphatic about the association between communication disorders and depression and learned helplessness (Seligman, 1975). Without exception, communication disorders have the potential for resulting in reactive depression for both the affected person and family members. With disorders that involve brain damage, concomitant depression may be brought about by faulty or disturbed patterns of normal neural transmission. Finally, some clients may have come to their present disorder already depressed. Nevertheless, it is essential to recognize that counselors in communication disorders lack the technical skills and the credentials to treat depression, either behaviorally or pharmacologically. But because depression is so likely to co-occur with the catastrophic problems we deal with, it is extremely important for us to be highly sensitive to problems that forecast it. The *Diagnostic and Statistical Manual of Mental Disorders*, 4th edition (DSM-IV) (American

Psychiatric Association, 1994), notes the following indicators as characteristic of depression: mood disorders, lack of zest, unexplained weight loss, sleeping problems, psychomotor problems, excessive fatigue, feelings of worthlessness, and statements of futility. When these indicators are present, the ethical responsibility of the SLP-A is to state relevant concerns directly, make appropriate referrals, and provide adequate follow-up regarding implementation of recommendations.

## Organization of the Rest of the Book

As noted earlier, Chapter 2 provides an introduction to positive psychology, which is the theoretical heart of this book's approach to communication counseling. Chapter 3 concerns clinical skills and specific techniques. The next four chapters focus specifically on counseling in communication disorders. They are developed according to a lifespan perspective. Thus, counseling in the context of communication problems emerging in infancy and early childhood is the first of these lifespan-oriented chapters (Chapter 4). Its focus is on working with parents and primary caregivers, in keeping with the principle that counseling without family "buy-in" will have only limited effectiveness. Counseling issues with older children and adolescents and their parents are addressed in Chapter 5.

Chapters 6 and 7 focus on adults. Chapter 6 concerns disorders whose natural progression is toward improvement (e.g., stroke, traumatic brain injury in adults, hearing disorders). Individual and group work is discussed for both individuals who have such disorders and their significant others. Chapter 7 concerns disorders whose natural progression is toward deterioration (e.g., Alzheimer's disease, Parkinson's disease). Chapter 8 presents some templates for workshops in resilience and optimism that can be adapted for use with families across the age span. Chapter 9, a gift from the pen of noted authority Stan Goldberg, provides insights into counseling for dying patients—an area that is virtually unmentioned in our field, yet one in which practitioners increasingly find themselves.

The "clinical" chapters are somewhat similarly ordered. Each chapter is organized to address issues that are unique in terms of the relevant information and counseling needs. Some attention also is given to both individual and group work. As noted previously, valuing stories and illness narratives is a critical part of the counseling process, so each chapter includes real stories about real problems providing everyday examples of a successful, positive, resilient outcome. Finally, each clinical chapter includes relevant learning exercises and formats for clinicians to use as practice. These exercises come mostly from my experiences in teaching communication counseling to graduate students.[3]

Other specific issues in communication counseling not covered in this book include counseling adult children of aging, communicatively impaired parents; counseling adults considering cochlear implants; and counseling elderly parents who have raised their children with chronic disabilities and communication disorders to adulthood. Of note, the principles embodied in the "wellness" approach to counseling are relevant to such issues as well and can be straightforwardly applied in appropriate instances.

Counseling skills cannot be learned effectively by reading about them. Rather, they are best learned through practice in constrained and nurturing environments, and through growing self-knowledge and introspection on the part of the learner. It is particularly critical for the SLP-A to think through personally experienced counseling moments and to evaluate them in ways suggested in this text.

The book's organization is based on the following assumptions. First, although a set of overarching principles is outlined for communication counseling, certain principles have more importance at some stages of the lifespan than at others. Such age specificity is a good reason for taking a lifespan approach. Furthermore, it seems unnecessary to differentiate a set of counseling principles aimed at specific problems. Principles that apply to counseling the parents of an at-risk infant (for example, helping them to become maximally resilient) will apply across a wide range of disorders. Thus, each chapter presents a few disorders as focal points, but the relevant techniques and skills have implications for the management of many other related disorders. These "focus disorders" are highly representative of the broader class of disorders that share their basic characteristics. Skilled clinicians rely on information concerning the facts of a given disorder, on community resources, and on the Internet. Such information itself is not inherent in the counseling process, but counseling certainly depends on it.

---

[3]I also am grateful to Michael Chial, PhD, and Michael Flahive, PhD, for providing guidance here.

# The Formalities

Finally, it is necessary to discuss the formalities of counseling for our professions. The most important ones are differences between group and individual counseling, the timing of counseling, and its intensity; these are discussed briefly next.

## Group and Individual Counseling

A natural inclination is to relegate *group counseling* and *individual counseling* to two separate, mutually exclusive categories, each of which is restricted to use in specific circumstances or for specific clients. This view is difficult to justify, however. Both modes are effective, and they can even be undertaken simultaneously.

My own clinical experience bears this out. Along with my commitment to shared expertise, I am inclined to favor group counseling. I like the notion of many experts in a room. Short-term discussion groups and workshops for families concerning specific disorders provide an opportunity to promote and foster shared stories and problem solving. Skill-focused workshops on topics such as developing resilience or learning effective parenting techniques are excellent venues for sharing informational aspects of the counseling process.

Alternatively, there is undeniable value in one-on-one interactions as well, but much of this work, as mentioned earlier, occurs at the outset or conclusion of more direct intervention, or is nestled into such sessions.

## Timing and Intensity of Counseling

Whether it is with individuals or groups, counseling should begin in the earliest phases of treatment, when it is most needed. This is true across the age spectrum, from parents' initial recognition that their child is at risk, to the early days following a stroke or a diagnosis of Alzheimer's disease. As mentioned earlier, providing information is just one of the functions of counseling, particularly early on. It also is important to remember that support and reassurance, as well as information, will continue to be needed as life with a problem is lived, but that the intensity of those needs should diminish. Thus, counseling often will occur in those counseling moments as described. Finally, a point worth repeating is that counseling is more than just a set of skills to be practiced with clients; it also incorporates an attitude of perceptiveness, respect, and sensitivity that permeates every aspect of every clinical interaction.

## Conclusions

This chapter provides an overview of a principled approach to communication counseling with a somewhat different focus from that of the more traditional approach. Although the SLP-A may view a leap into this relative unknown as a risky undertaking, the novel principles and techniques presented are neither untested nor without application in other fields.

In the following poem, the rewards of maintaining an openness to change, despite its risks, are well illustrated:

The Guest House

This being human is a guest house.
Every morning a new arrival.

A joy, a depression, a meanness,
some momentary awareness comes
as an unexpected visitor.

Welcome and entertain them all!
Even if they're a crowd of sorrows,
Who violently sweep your house
empty of its furniture.

Still, treat each guest honorably.
He may be cleaning you out
for some new delight.

The dark moment, the shame, the malice,
Meet them at the door laughing,
and invite them in.

Be grateful for whoever comes,
Because each has been sent
as a guide from beyond.

Jalal al-Din Rumi
*The Essential Rumi: Translations by Coleman Barks with John Moyne*, 1995. Reprinted with permission from HarperCollins.

## References

American Psychiatric Association. (1994). *Diagnostic and statistical manual of mental disorders* (4th ed.). Washington, DC: Author.

American Speech-Language-Hearing Association. (2001). *Scope of practice in speech-language pathology*. Available at http://www.asha.org

American Speech-Language-Hearing Association. (2004). *Scope of practice in audiology*. Available at http://www.asha.org

Barnes, C., Mercer, G., & Shakespeare, T. (1999). *Exploring disability: A sociological introduction*. Cambridge, UK: Polity.

Chodron, P. (2001). *The places that scare you: A guide to fearlessness in difficult times*. Boston: Shambhala.

Coles, R. (1989). *The call of stories: Teaching and the moral imagination*. Boston: Houghton Mifflin.

Frank, A. (1995). *The wounded storyteller: Body, illness and ethics*. Chicago: University of Chicago Press.

Goldberg, S. (2006). Shedding your fears: Bedside etiquette for dying patients. *Topics in Stroke Rehabilitation, 13*, 63–67.

Haidt, J. (2006). *The happiness hypothesis: Finding modern truth in ancient wisdom*. New York: Basic Books.

Hinckley, J. (2006). Finding messages in bottles: Successful living with aphasia as revealed through personal narrative. *Topics in Stroke Rehabilitation, 13*, 25–36.

Kabat-Zinn, J. (2005). *Full catastrophe living. Using the wisdom of your body and mind to face stress, pain, and illness* (15th anniversary ed.). New York: Delta.

Kazantsakis, N. (1996). *Zorba the Greek*. New York: Scribner.

Kleinman, A. (1988). *The illness narratives: Suffering healing and the human condition*. New York: Basic Books.

Kübler-Ross, E. (1969). *On death and dying*. New York: Macmillan.

Lomas, J., Pickard, L., Bester, S., Elbard, H., Findlayson, A., & Zoghabib, C. (1989). The Communicative Effectiveness Index: Development and psychometric evaluation of functional communication measure for adult aphasia. *Journal of Speech and Hearing Disorders, 54,* 113–124.

Oliver, J. (1996). *Understanding disability: From theory to practice.* Basingstroke: Macmillan.

Peterson, C. (2006). *A primer in positive psychology.* New York: Oxford University Press.

Ram Dass. (2000). *Still here,* p. 185. New York: Riverhead.

Reivich, K., & Shatté, A. (2002). *The resilience factor.* New York: Broadway Books.

Robbins, T. (1980). *Still life with woodpecker.* New York: Bantam.

Rogers, C. (1995). *Client-centered therapy: Its current practice, implications and theory.* Philadelphia: Trans-Atlantic.

Rumi, J. D. (1995). The guest house. In *The essential Rumi* (C. Barks & J. Moyne, Trans.). San Francisco: HarperSanFrancisco.

Seligman, M. E. P. (1975). *Helplessness: On depression, development and death.* San Francisco: W. H. Freeman.

Seligman, M. E. P. (1991). *Learned optimism.* New York: Alfred A. Knopf.

Seligman, M. (2002). *Authentic happiness.* New York: Free Press.

Snyder, C., & Lopez, S. (2005). *Handbook of positive psychology.* New York: Oxford University Press.

Webster, E. (1977). *Counseling with parents of handicapped children: Guidelines for improving communication.* New York: Grune & Stratton.

Webster, E., & Newhoff, M. (1981). Intervention with families of communicatively impaired adults. In D. S. Beasley & G. A. Davis (Eds.). *Aging: Communication processes and disorders.* New York: Grune & Stratton.

World Health Organization. (2001). *International classification of functioning, disability and health.* Geneva: Author.

# Chapter 2

# POSITIVE PSYCHOLOGY: IN BRIEF

Sam Schmidt is a quadriplegic former race car driver (who sustained his life-altering injury while racing). On announcing the development of the Sam Schmidt Paralysis Foundation, devoted to research, funding, and advocacy for persons with spinal cord injuries and other neurological disorders, he commented:

> "If I didn't have something like this going on, I'd probably be depressed. I'd be thinking about what I can't do instead of what I can do."
>
> "The way I look at it, before I was hurt, I was one of 100 drivers making a living at the top level of motor sports. Now, I'm an ex-Indy-car driver, who's paralyzed. There's only one of me." (Auto Racing: Ex-Driver Becomes a Driving Force, 2005)

This uniquely positive outlook is evident to those around him: "Ritchie Hearn, who drove one of Schmidt's cars in the 2005 Indy 500, noted: 'One of his (Sam's) biggest things is showing people they have hope'" (Auto Racing: Ex-Driver Becomes a Driving Force, 2005).

## What Is Positive Psychology?

To say that Martin E. P. Seligman and his colleagues at the end of the 20th century launched the positive psychology movement is an exaggeration. Many spiritual leaders (start with Confucius) and psychologists (include Abraham Maslow and Carl Rogers) set the stage. Yet it is relatively easy to trace its current ascendance to Seligman's presidential address to the American Psychological Association (Seligmann, 1999) and its further explication by Seligman and Csikszenthmihalyi, (2000). Earlier, Seligman, with Stephen Maier and then Christopher Peterson, described the now-familiar concept of "learned helplessness" (Maier & Seligman, 1976; Peterson, Maier, & Seligman, 1993) and pioneered the concept of "learned optimism" (Seligman, 1990). In his 1999 address, Seligman charted a new territory for the scientific study of psychology. He accurately noted that since the end of World War II, clinical psychology had shifted the bulk of its attention away from the task of making people's lives more fulfilling to the task of curing mental illness. Seligman contended that to be truly comprehensive, the discipline of psychology also had to concern itself with describing and enhancing mental *wellness*.

Depression is more prevalent in the United States than it was some 50 years ago, and its age at onset has decreased so that it is now a disorder that disproportionately affects American teenagers, rather than persons facing middle age. Lewinsohn, Hops, Roberts, and Seeley (1993) noted that one in five adolescents can be expected to have a major depressive episode during high school. This increase in prevalence among the young has occurred despite the development of more effective treatments ranging from the pharmacological to the behavioral. Thus there exists the paradox of more effective treatment yet greater pervasiveness of depression. Why?

Seligman's contention is that psychology and its related professions have failed to attend to issues concerning relative mental health, contentment, satisfaction, and the ability to enhance quality of life in favor of concentrating on ways to lessen mental illness. In the process, both scientists and the broader Western lay community have become erroneously convinced that *happiness* is the opposite of *depression*. The truth is that the opposite of *depressed* is just *not depressed*. Being not depressed is far from being happy, the stated goal of most individuals, including those who undergo formal psychotherapy for depression.

What was needed, Seligman further contended, was not that psychology abandon its concern with mental illness, but rather that it also focus a considerable amount of attention on the intensive and systematic study of what is *right* in human behavior. Scientific psychology also should include the study of what is positive and how happiness can be increased. Furthermore, psychology should focus on how to help people build and increase their strengths and how to flourish, rather than concentrating specifically on how they can reduce and eradicate weaknesses. As a result of scholarly and research attention since 1999, positive psychology has enjoyed remarkable and growing influence worldwide. For a few relevant and important examples, see recent works by Aspinwall and Staudinger (2004), Gilbert (2006), Haidt (2006), Peterson (2006), Peterson and Seligman (2004), Seligman (2003), Seligman (2005), and Snyder and Lopez (2005).

Clinical applications have been well described not only for professionals but also for lay audiences. Perhaps the most influential example of this work is the book *Authentic Happiness* (Seligman, 2002) and the websites it has spawned, particularly http://www. authentichappiness.org and http://www.reflectivehappiness.com. Attesting to the growth of this movement, the University of Pennsylvania recently initiated a master's degree training program in positive psychology geared to training psychologists, life coaches, and other allied health professionals to this aspect of the discipline of psychology.

## Positive Psychology and Disability

This renaissance of interest in what is "right" about people already has brought about a number of relevant observations, described in detail later in the chapter. Here, some reasons why positive psychology has particular resonance for counseling individuals with communication disabilities are reviewed. First, conditions such as difficult early life experiences (Roberts, Brown, Johnson, & Reinke, 2002), physical disability (Elliott, Kurylo, & Rivera, 2002), and aging

(Vaillant, 2002) do not necessarily have negative consequences, as has typically been assumed. Second, it is possible to describe and measure human strengths. Third, to some large degree it is possible to use personal strengths to increase overall life satisfaction and happiness. Finally, and most pertinent to communication counseling, people can be helped to develop resilience and optimism (Reivich & Shatté, 2002), as well as new forms of positive behaviors (Fredrickson, 2001; Fredrickson & Losada, 2005) that may enrich their lives. Skills such as these probably are crucial for everyday people to live successfully (that is, fully) in the wake of catastrophic events.

Positive psychology's emphasis on wellness and full living resonates with abandonment of sole reliance on a disease model in "helping" professions such as speech pathology and audiology. Positive psychology also appears to fit comfortably with a number of other recent issues and developments pertinent to communication counseling. These include the social model of disability, the expanded idea of who the experts are, the rising role of the consumer in defining the delivery of health care, and the growing respect for many forms of alternative medicine and approaches to counseling and coaching.

## Some Tenets of Positive Psychology

This section presents a brief overview of some basic tenets of positive psychology, with an emphasis on those that seem particularly pertinent to counseling in communication disorders. (The description of the latter emphasis bears some similarity to a fifteen-minute lecture on "Freud's Contributions to Western Thought"!) For readers interested in further exploration, the extensive bibliography should be useful. Many of these concepts are visited in more detail later in the book as well. Because today's positive psychology has benefited to some degree by its concurrence with the "Age of the Internet," the bibliography contains references to a number of relevant websites, as well as books and articles. The following overview uses examples from clinical cases involving communication disorders to illustrate the importance of the three themes of positive psychology. The themes, of course, are larger and more pervasive than the simple examples.

## Positive Psychology Is as Concerned with Discovering Strength as it is with Modulating Weakness

For communication counseling, an equal focus on maximizing strength and on modulating or compensating for weakness means specifically that it is critical to look at not only the devastation and malfunctioning brought about by a communication disorder but beyond it, to the strengths that the affected person possesses. Clinicians must help their clients to discover and then to capitalize on their true strengths,[1] as well as to develop nascent ones. Here's an example of how this might work:

> Surely, Adama and Evan, who have just become parents of a child with Down syndrome, are devastated by this fact. Their catastrophe must be acknowledged. But what *strengths* do Adama and Evan possess that can be counted on to help them develop the resilience and optimism necessary to raise their baby successfully? Is Adama brave? Is Evan intellectually curious? Does either have a sense of humor and playfulness? How can these or other strengths be harnessed to help them manage the care and planning their Down syndrome child will need?

## Positive Psychology Focuses Equally on Building on the Best Things in Life and on Repairing the Worst

One goal of communication counseling that follows from the principle of equal emphasis on building and repair in life is that we play a part in helping parents, persons with disorders, and families to live as fully as possible despite their catastrophe. Here is a pertinent example:

> Joe and Sue had just begun their carefully planned and anticipated retirement life together when Sue had a major stroke that left her with moderately severe Broca's aphasia and right hemiplegia. It is crucial to hear from both of them how their best-laid retirement plans were left in ruins, and to honor the

---

[1]Measurement of strengths and virtues is discussed later in the chapter.

problems they face. However, the focus for the long haul (after suitable healing time) should be on what is still good. What pieces of their plans can be salvaged? What still works for them? For example, under these changed circumstances, how can they now take advantage of and maximize visits with their grandchildren? Can a travel agent experienced in working with disabled individuals be hired to help in future travel planning? Can an architect be found to modify the vacation home they designed years ago? How do Sue and Joe approach the architect and the travel agent?

## Positive Psychology Is Equally Concerned with Fulfilling the Lives of Normal People and with Healing Pathologic Conditions

A key assumption in the counseling approach presented in this book is that basically normal people are likely to be the recipients of communication counseling. This assumption has powerful repercussions for us as clinicians in the ways we approach clients. Thus, we do not have to be experts in pathological denial, in transference, or in any of the traditions and variants of Freudian psychotherapy. We do have to recognize such problems when we see them, and to make appropriate referrals, but they will not dominate our interactions. The notion that we deal with generally normal people in catastrophic situations should normalize *us*, and help us to ask the right questions, listen appropriately, and provide wise, pertinent professional advice.

Some of our clients *will* have psychopathologic conditions, of course, and we have to be experts at recognizing such conditions and making appropriate referrals. People with longstanding bipolar disease, for example, are not immune to developing a communication disorder, or to giving birth to a child who has one. Also, as previously noted, reactive depression, particularly for adults with neurogenic disorders, is quite common. But our own counseling job is much more strongly focused on normality in catastrophic situations than it is on psychopathology. The focus is on "What's right with you?" rather than on "What's wrong with you?" and how our clients can use what is right about them to help them to manage their current catastrophes. Here's an example of how it might work:

Five-year-old Sean's parents are not particularly concerned that he is "slow in talking." Sean is an only child. His parents can understand most of what he says; he communicates "just fine" at home and has good social relationships in his kindergarten. The only reason they have come for this evaluation is that Sean's teacher is very worried about what is going to happen to him in first grade. The evaluation reveals that Sean is a delightful little boy, very sociable and outgoing, but his speech is largely unintelligible. He shows remarkable ingenuity in communicating nonetheless. His hearing is normal.

He gestures, points, drags folks around, and is extremely responsive to prompts from others, suggesting minimal comprehension problems. Are these parents denying the potential severity of the situation? Will they benefit from counseling to help them develop insight into Sean's phonological problems? Such counseling probably is not a very effective use of their (or the counselor's or Sean's) time. Sean needs direct speech intervention, and his family needs to learn about language development and how they can harness Sean's strengths, as well as their own, to help with this process. That is, they need information and some understanding of the importance of their involvement in direct speech therapy. They need to be added to Sean's therapy team. Even from this brief summary, some of Sean's strengths, as well as those of his parents, are pretty easy to find. These strengths will be the counterweights to his problems and as such should facilitate therapy.

## Routes to Happiness

The three routes to happiness identified by Seligman are (1) the "pleasant life," (2) the "engaged life," and (3) the "meaningful life." The notion of such pathways is not new. Seligman points out that what he calls "pillars" of authentic happiness have concerned philosophy and religion for centuries (Seligman, 2002). These three routes (also called "pillars" in the following discussion) can be seen as the three legs of a triangle—metaphorically, perhaps a three-legged stool. Although for most people, a perfect balance probably is not achievable, a triangular structure is notable for stability and strength. So even though an unbalanced stool is hard to sit on, all three of its components contribute significantly to a cohesive and recognizable shape. It really does not matter how you visualize this concept, except to remember that happiness and well-being can be thought of as having three critical interacting facets, each contributing (not necessarily equally) to personal contentment and flourishing. Each of these facets is described next.

## Positive Emotion: The Pleasant Life

There are three aspects to the pleasant life. The first concerns the past and its satisfactions and the contentment that comes from recollecting these memories. The second addresses living fully in the present moment. The third involves anticipation, looking forward to the future.

### The Past Pleasant Life

The "past pleasant life" depends on positive and fulfilling recollections. For example, Joe and Sue (of the earlier example) report that in the past, they have enjoyed cooking together, seeing foreign movies, and taking languorous vacations in the Caribbean. Could they develop a collection of their best recipes as a legacy for their children? Can they use subtitled films to work on Sue's reading? What could now be gained by putting together a long-planned scrapbook of their previous vacation on Eleuthera or Jamaica, possibly permitting them to savor their time spent relaxing there in earlier years? These notions probably can be built into direct therapy, of course, and not simply reserved for the communication counseling parts of treatment.

### Present Pleasures

The second aspect of the pleasant life concerns the pleasures of "present living." Included here are the satisfactions derived from activities as diverse as eating, talking with friends, and having satisfying sexual experiences. Little things, perhaps less obvious, contribute to the pleasant life—perhaps a pet's enthusiastic greeting at the end of the workday. The burdens of a handicapped child or the stress resulting from living with a partner with Alzheimer's disease can clearly intrude on present pleasures.

### Pleasant Life in the Future

The third aspect of the pleasant life concerns the future. To achieve a "pleasant life in the future," the key is to develop optimism and resilience; this is the basis of some techniques and exercises we may practice ourselves and encourage our clients to practice. How shall we face the future? What current strengths can be mustered? What new skills can be learned to increase the ability to face what is ahead with flexibility, grace, bravery, and hope? How can we help our clients to learn them?

The pleasant life is perhaps the easiest of the three routes to happiness to connect with. It's important, however, not to equate the pleasant life with "happiness." In fact, some people who have few overtly positive emotions nevertheless are living fulfilled and happy lives, largely as a result of their engagement and their devotion to the meaningful life. Some well-known religious figures such as the Dalai Lama or Mother Teresa come to mind, but most of us also know some less renowned examples. These second and third pillars probably are ultimately more important to a broad conceptualization of happiness that includes fulfillment and flourishing, a life well and satisfactorily lived. These are discussed next.

## The Engaged Life

As conceptualized by Seligman, the engaged life is the second pillar of happiness. All of us have, at some time, been so absorbed in what we were doing that time slipped away and we failed to realize that we missed making a previously arranged phone call or forgot to take the cake from the oven. Sometimes these experiences are annoying or frustrating. But there is also undeniable pleasure to be found in absorption. And for most of us, the *totally* pleasurable experiences of losing oneself in a tennis or video game or in a walk on the beach in the moonlight greatly outnumber those episodes involving burned cake. Truly engaging experiences such as those just described constitute the essence of "flow" as described by Csikszentmihalyi (1990, 1997). The engaged life, from the viewpoint of experienced meditators, seems to be kin to being "in the moment" (Chodron, 2000; Kabat-Zinn, 1994). Haidt (2006) calls flow "the state of total immersion in a task that is challenging yet closely matched to one's abilities" (p. 95).

This temporary loss of a sense of time may be difficult to appreciate because often we are unaware of it when it occurs. But for artists and athletes, this sense of engagement and flow is unquestioned. For example, consider the samurai archer, who is at one with his bow—or, perhaps closer to home, Peyton Manning on a really good day. Flow matters for more ordinary people as well, even though they may not be specifically aware of its value.

Unfortunately, flow and the engaged life may be among the first casualties for people who are beginning the process of dealing with the downside of their catastrophes. The mother of a child with disabilities who mourns the loss of time for herself may feel guilty about missing her time alone. She is unaware of how important this pillar of happiness is. I recently heard a despairing description of such loss, as told by Mrs. J, the spouse of an aphasic man. Mrs. J perceived Mr. J as totally demanding of her energies as she helped him to carry out his prescribed after-stroke regimen: "I have to do everything, go everywhere with him. I'm not even alone when I'm sound asleep!" Mrs. J lamented the loss of personal control over the pace of her own life and, no doubt, the loss of flow. Jon Lyon (1998) notes about flow that

> . . . all people need frequent and predictable periods in their lives when the actual act of participating in life dominates self-awareness, self-consciousness, even awareness of reward! . . . the captivating nature of simply "doing" the activity that causes its initiator to forget entirely about self, time, or outcome (p. 222).

In communication counseling, we must pay serious attention to ways of reestablishing engagement and flow in the lives of our clients and their families. For example, it is easier to find absorption in an activity that harnesses personal strengths. This is an important reason to identify such strengths.

## The Meaningful Life

Seligman's conception of the meaningful life is simply "using your strengths and virtues in the service of something larger than you are" (Seligman, 2002, p. 263). He further notes that this outside responsibility could be to anything from family concerns, to allegiance to the Rotary Club, to the strict observance of religious practices. In the days following Hurricane Katrina, in the midst of reports concerning the devastation and horror in Louisiana, Mississippi, and Alabama, many instances of incredible bravery and outpouring of money, help, and services to the hurricane's victims also occurred. This example was found on an anonymous website: Greg Henderson, a pathologist in New Orleans, described the overwhelming difficulty he experienced in providing medical service there. "We are under martial law so return to our homes is impossible," he wrote in an e-mail message on August 31, 2005. "I don't know how long it will be and this is my greatest fear. Despite it all, this is a soul-edifying experience."

Here is another example, pieced together from a National Public Radio (NPR) broadcast at about the same time: The town of Lake Providence, Louisiana, a crushingly poor community of 5000 in East Carroll Parish, opened its arms to refugees from Katrina's aftermath. One such refugee told a BBC reporter that after he revisited New Orleans to reclaim what was left of his life there, he planned to return and to live in Lake Providence. When the reporter asked why, he responded, "Because good people live here." When one of those good local residents was asked how she explained the citizens' outpouring of care, fund-raising, and support, she replied, "We are poor people here. We know what this feels like."

In the case of families of children with communication disorders and families and individuals who have incurred them later in life, three themes are implicit in the foregoing examples: (1) What commitments to the meaningful life were in place before the catastrophe? (2) How can they be optimized? (3) Can new commitments emerge as the result of this potentially transformative experience?

This cursory look at the values and principles of positive psychology is intended to lead the reader to further reading, particularly of the sources referred to in the bibliography. Throughout the course of this book, the reader is encouraged to visit the various websites related to authentic happiness and positive psychology. To find out about the "shape of your own triangle" so to speak, you can visit, register, and log onto the following websites:

- http://www.authentichappiness.org
- www.authentichappiness.sas.upenn.edu

These websites furnish a number of free tests that can be useful in developing self-knowledge and understanding to use in counseling, or to which the counselor may want to refer clients. Pertinent to this topic, Christopher Peterson's brief life satisfaction measure, called Approaches to Happiness, is available on the authentic happiness website. It provides you with your own profile relative to the three pillars and permits you to compare yourself with a larger sample of people who share some of your demographics.

## Learning Your Strengths and Helping Others to Learn Theirs

Setting the boundaries on what psychological happiness and well-being might look like is an important step in exploring the basics of positive psychology. Also at issue, however, is developing a style of living in the world that capitalizes on using one's own strengths. Western culture encourages people to know their limitations, to seek self-improvement, and to live within their constraints. (Consider that as of 2007, www.amazon.com listed almost 30,000 titles under the heading of personal growth, including one on writing self-help books.)

Far less attention has been given to recognizing personal strengths and virtues and capitalizing on them, or using them to shore up some less well-honed traits. A useful guide for finding personal strengths is the Values in Action (VIA) assessment available through the Authentic Happiness website mentioned earlier. This measure, developed by Peterson and Seligman, is the product of a principled attempt to provide a foundation in psychology for the scientific study of character and grew out of their book *Character Strengths and Virtues: A Classification and Handbook* (2004). Seligman refers to this book as an "un-DSM."[2] Peterson and Seligman, to some degree following the template that was used to develop the DSM, have produced a "Manual of the Sanities" (Peterson &

---

[2]DSM is the *Diagnostic and Statistical Manual of Mental Disorders*, which is a widely disseminated manual of definitions of disorders of mental health, and information on how to assess and, in some instances, treat them. The *Manual* currently is in its fourth revised edition (DSM-IV-TR), with a fifth edition (DSM-V) in the planning stages.

Seligman, 2004, p. 3). The authors first explored a vast number of resources, consulting a large pool of eminent authorities in human behavior and combing the world's philosophies, religions, literatures, films, and so on, for possible contributions to a list of character strengths. Next, they developed criteria for reducing this large data pool into a more manageable list of character strengths and virtues. At this step, they again sought input from their group of authorities. What finally emerged is a classification system designed to exemplify core properties of character, applicable across cultures and religions.[3] A list of these character strengths appears as Box 2.1. Please be aware that this list is really a "work in progress" amenable to change and modification over time.

Note that the list comprises six core moral virtues recognized by the world's religions, and thought to be universal. These moral virtues are temperance, transcendence, wisdom and knowledge, courage, humanity, and justice. Listed under each are the specific traits that address the core moral virtues. Twenty-four are identified, each a trait for people to consider in relation to themselves as they take the VIA to find their strengths. No one will find that he or she is blessed with all 24; in fact, the VIA concentrates on an individual's five most prominent ones, referred to as "signature strengths." Peterson and Seligman (2004, p.18) note that such strengths (or personal traits) are the stuff of the *real me*, "the strengths that one owns, celebrates, frequently exercises. And most of us know what some of them are."

A cornerstone of this book is that counselor-clinicians need to know themselves. (More on this precept is presented in the next chapter.) To apply positive psychology to communication counseling, it is necessary to become familiar with its exercises and approaches, an exploration that furnishes common ground for both counselors and their clients. Doing the exercises and taking the assessment test also may be of direct personal benefit. Therefore, self-administration of the VIA (available on the aforementioned websites) to get a blueprint of personal signature strengths is a useful undertaking for all SLP-As. After completion of the VIA and review of the results, illustrating for a client how to use them as fully as possible is easier. Relevant questions to ponder include

---

[3]A highly recommended distillation of character strengths and virtues can be found in Peterson's *A Primer in Positive Psychology* (2006).

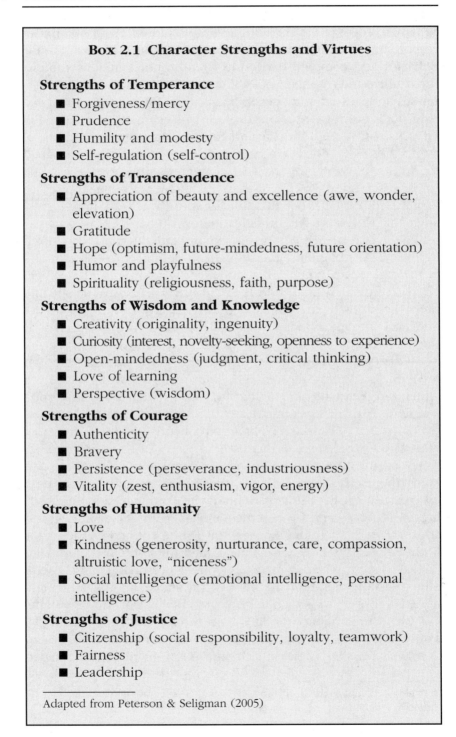

## Box 2.1 Character Strengths and Virtues

**Strengths of Temperance**
- Forgiveness/mercy
- Prudence
- Humility and modesty
- Self-regulation (self-control)

**Strengths of Transcendence**
- Appreciation of beauty and excellence (awe, wonder, elevation)
- Gratitude
- Hope (optimism, future-mindedness, future orientation)
- Humor and playfulness
- Spirituality (religiousness, faith, purpose)

**Strengths of Wisdom and Knowledge**
- Creativity (originality, ingenuity)
- Curiosity (interest, novelty-seeking, openness to experience)
- Open-mindedness (judgment, critical thinking)
- Love of learning
- Perspective (wisdom)

**Strengths of Courage**
- Authenticity
- Bravery
- Persistence (perseverance, industriousness)
- Vitality (zest, enthusiasm, vigor, energy)

**Strengths of Humanity**
- Love
- Kindness (generosity, nurturance, care, compassion, altruistic love, "niceness")
- Social intelligence (emotional intelligence, personal intelligence)

**Strengths of Justice**
- Citizenship (social responsibility, loyalty, teamwork)
- Fairness
- Leadership

Adapted from Peterson & Seligman (2005)

the following: "How do I feel when I am using a top strength?" "How can I use my strengths in my professional life?" "How can I engage my strengths further, and what benefits might they confer to my clients?"

# Evidence

Many of the claims made by positive psychology have been addressed by relevant research. This section does not attempt to review all of the findings but rather presents appropriate examples to illustrate their breadth. Two areas are central to the practice of communication counseling focused on wellness:

1. The importance of optimism for developing and maintaining physical and psychological health and well-being
2. The idea that happiness and optimism can be increased, which is central to the counseling model presented in this book. Although they are interrelated, they are discussed separately in this section.

## The Importance of Optimism and Resilience for Authentic Happiness[4]

As a prerequisite to considering its relevance in counseling, an explicit definition of *resilience* is necessary. Resilience is not just interior toughness, nor is it the ability to forge ahead no matter what, alone and against overwhelming, perhaps invincible, odds. Few would deny that Lance Armstrong is a poster child for

---

[4]This section relies heavily on my notes from the course "Authentic Happiness Master Class," conducted by Martin E. P. Seligman (May–October 2004) via Internet and telephone, and on the details of conversations during the course with members of a small group of fellow students facilitated by Karen Reivich, PhD. This latter group still flourishes through its weekly interactions, and the input of its members is gratefully acknowledged both here and in the more formal Acknowledgments section. I am specifically grateful to Dr. Reivich for sharing with me her notes on resilience and optimism for lectures she presented in the University of Pennsylvania's Master's Program in Positive Psychology (2006).

resilience, defined most rigorously in this way. But resilience also consists of factors that can be more prosaically embodied for most other people, who probably were never destined to win even a single neighborhood tricycle race. Werner and Smith (1982) describe resilience simply as the quality that enables people to thrive despite adversity. This definition is expanded on by Peterson (2006) and is operationalized in many activities adapted from Reivich and Shatté (2002), presented later in this book. Here, the focus is on a study reported by Charney (2005), who investigated American servicemen who survived imprisonment for six to eight years during the Vietnam War. They found that servicemen who did not develop post-traumatic stress disorder (PTSD) exhibited the characteristics that are presented in Box 2.2. A reasonable assumption is that the subjects of this research constitute a random sample of American servicemen, not supermen. But they were resilient, and resilience comprises these characteristics. In the words of Ann Masten (2001), such resilience probably is "ordinary magic." If it is a teachable skill, consider what it may offer to parents and families with communication disorders.

Many studies have examined the relationship between the qualities of optimism and resilience and mental and physical health. In the context of physical health, research has shown, for example, that optimists live longer than pessimists (Maruta, Colli-

---

### Box 2.2 Qualities and Factors
### Associated with Resilience in POWs

- Optimism
- Altruism—helping others reduce stress
- Having an enduring set of beliefs or a moral compass
- Faith and spirituality
- Humor
- Having a role model
- Having social supports
- Being able to leave one's comfort zones (facing fear)
- Having a mission or meaning in life
- Having some training in mastering challenges

Adapted from Charney (2005)

gan, Malinchoc, & Offord, 2000), have healthier immune functions (Segerstrom, Taylor, Kemeny, & Fahey, 1998), and recover more quickly from bypass surgery (Fitzgerald, Tennen, Affleck, & Pransky 1993). Optimistic students visit their doctors less frequently and have fewer physical illnesses (Peterson & Bossio, 1991).

Similarly, optimists appear to be mentally healthier. A brief sampling of the relevant research supports this: Optimists are less likely to get depressed (Chang, 2000). Optimistic people have richer and more fulfilling social lives than pessimists (Diener & Seligman, 2002). Optimists age better than pessimists (Vaillant, 2002). That is, they have more satisfying relationships and are healthier and more contented than less optimistic people. Hollon and associates (2005) suggest that in cognitive therapy, one mediator of outcome is increases in optimism. Reivich, Gillham, Shatté, and Seligman (2006) found that in children, optimism also mediates the likelihood and degree of depression. According to Seligman (1998), optimistic insurance agents even sell more insurance.

This is not to say that there are no negative consequences to a high level of optimism. Taylor and Brown (1988) have noted that mentally healthier people tend to overestimate the degree of their environmental control, see themselves in a perhaps overly positive light, and are sometimes unrealistically optimistic about the future.

Reivich and Shatté (2002) caution against such *cockeyed optimism* and instead suggest the concept of "realistic optimism" (i.e., maintaining a positive outlook without denying observable and verifiable facts, or ignoring negative aspects). Schneider (2001) discusses the "real world" issue of situations that permit latitude in how events are to be interpreted (she refers to them as having "fuzzy meaning"). She points out that denying or downplaying facts is neither helpful nor adaptive, and that optimism and pessimism both require caution and tempering. Aspinwall and colleagues (2000, 2001) also suggest that optimists must not ignore negative information but rather use it as a barometer for changing strategies and as the basis for improving their performances. Nevertheless, the evidence supports the importance of optimism and resilience in flourishing and living well.

### Positive Emotions and Flourishing.

The role of the positive emotions (e.g., love, hope, trust, awe, enjoyment) and their importance in the good life were explored in the pioneering work of Barbara Fredrickson and her colleagues at the University of Michigan. Fredrickson's seminal contribution to the field has been to begin the process of explaining why the ability to experience positive emotion may be the basis of successful living, or flourishing, as many positive psychologists refer to thriving in a satisfying and meaningful life.

Specifically, Fredrickson and her colleagues have developed a theory called *broaden-and-build* (Fredrickson, 2001). In this theory, positive and negative emotions are distinctive and complementary.

Negative emotions (e.g., anger, fear, sadness) tend to narrow people's reactive abilities to those that have fostered survival. (Seligman refers to our "Pleistocene heritage" to describe them.) The "fight or flight" response is the primary example. Largely reactive (and not necessarily the subject of painstaking consideration, debate, and reconsideration), they are behavioral automatisms that have had an undeniable role in survival not only for our ancestors but also in many situations in the twenty-first century, such as the East Asian Tsunami, our own Hurricane Katrina, and the devastating earthquakes in Pakistan.

Positive emotions, on the other hand, "broaden an individual's momentary thought-action repertoire and undo the narrow psychological and physiological preparation for specific action" (Fredrickson, 1998). In the context of a wellness-based approach to counseling, broadened repertoires of actions include helping people to see the "big picture" and to help them to frame it in optimistic, positive nurturing terms.

Fredrickson's broaden-and-build theory posits that broadening provides a foundation for developing a person's strengths, including physical and intellectual strengths, as well as social and psychological ones. Fredrickson's hypothesis states that over time, positive emotions increase and become more extensive, consequential personal resources. Fredrickson's recent work with Losada (Fredrickson & Losada, 2005) looked at a large sample of subjects' reports of their experienced positive and negative emotions over 28 days. Using a nonlinear dynamic model, the investigators concluded that a certain ratio of positive to negative events was predictive of flourishing.

This ratio is important—in fact, it is very important. Specifically, Fredrickson and Losada found that flourishing (as well as positive emotion) results when positive experiences (even such simple things as receiving a compliment on one's work) and negative experiences (again, possibly as simple as hearing that one's work is sloppy) occur in about a 3:1 ratio, with the upper limit set at 12:1. This finding should give clinicians and counselors pause. We have been brought up on the notion that positive reinforcement is desirable, and Fredrickson and Losada's research to some degree substantiates this. But the negative consequences of overkill constitute just as important a finding. It is not hard to imagine that nondiscriminative overflows such as "great," wonderful," or "cool" become meaningless to most people when delivered at even a 10:1 ratio; as a result, broadening-and-building in the clinical context may fail to occur. ("Cheerleading" is neither broadening nor building.) These findings are particularly important for SLP-As if they aim to cultivate positive emotions in their clients to maximize health and well-being (Fredrickson, 2001).

## Exercises and Interventions: Evidence of Their Importance

Applied positive psychology incorporates many exercises and practices intended to illustrate particular points. These interventions also are learning experiences designed to teach new ways of thinking and new patterns of behavior. This book incorporates a number of the approaches that have been validated by research, as well as others (not necessarily from positive psychology), that are designed to enhance counseling skills. Box 2.3 describes five positive psychology interventions that were designed to increase individual happiness. These five have been evaluated for their efficacy (Seligman, Steen, Park, & Peterson, 2005).

Detailed instructions for carrying out these interventions can be found in *Authentic Happiness* (Seligman, 2002) and at the Reflective Happiness website. A few of them also are incorporated in later chapters.

Seligman and his colleagues made these exercises and a placebo control task available via the Internet and asked interested participants to practice the interventions according to the researchers' instructions. Randomly assigned to study and placebo conditions, individuals were tested before and then after participation and at 1 week after the post-test and then at 1, 3, and 6 months

---

### Box 2.3 Five Positive Psychology Interventions*

**Gratitude visit:** Write and then deliver a letter of gratitude to a person who has been very kind to you, but whom you have never properly thanked.

**Three good things in life:** Write down three things that went well each day for a week. Include what you did to bring this good thing about.

**You at your best:** Write about an instance in your life that shows you at your best. Review the story daily and consider which of your strengths was/were involved.

**Using signature strengths in a new way:** After taking the VIA and receiving feedback concerning signature strengths, use one of them in a new and different way every day for a week.[†]

**Identifying signature strengths:** Note your five most pronounced strengths, and use them more often for a week.

---

*Studied in Seligman, Steen, Park, & Peterson, 2005.

†A fine collection of ideas for implementing this intervention appears in Peterson's *A Primer in Positive Psychology* (2006, pp 159–162).

---

after the post-test using the Steen Happiness Index (SHI) and the Center for Epidemiological Studies Depression Scale (CES-D).[5] The assessments were self-administered at the website. A total of 411 subjects participated in all of the follow-up assessments. The interventions "using signature strengths in a new way" and "three good things in life" resulted in increased SHI scores and decreased CES-D scores, with effects continuing for the entire follow-up period. The "gratitude visit" intervention produced changes that persisted for one month. The "you at your best" and "identifying signature strengths" interventions resulted in positive but transient effects on SHI and CES-D scores. The placebo treatment of writing about early memories every night for 1 week also demonstrated positive, transient effects in control subjects.

---

[5]Both instruments are available on the Authentic Happiness website, and the CES-D also is available on the CES-D website. Lower scores on CES-D are better, incidentally.

An important finding of this study was that although subjects were asked to follow the protocol for only one week, a substantial number continued to practice the exercises. Subsequent analysis of subjects who continued the exercises provided strong evidence that those who continued to practice the interventions showed longer-term benefit.

Problems with this research range from self-selection of participants to lack of careful definition of participant characteristics. Nevertheless, it constitutes important work and provides justification for more widespread use of the interventions. SLP-As can use the exercises with family members without modification, although for communicatively disordered adults, relatively simple changes may be required. These interventions will be far more meaningful to the counselor if experienced personally, so all clinicians should perform the exercises themselves before asking their clients to do so.

Of note, precursors of these interventions, as well as a model for their use, have been influenced by work in cognitive behavioral therapy (CBT) for treatment of depression (Beck, 1973; Beck, Rush, Shaw, & Emery, 1979, Young, Weinberger & Beck,2001. CBT is an approach to intervention that is rooted in reality and committed to change. CBT traditionally uses various behavioral exercises and interventions geared to helping depressed persons learn to reframe their thinking into healthier ways, and to put this new thinking into practice. A number of studies have supported the use of CBT in the treatment of depression and other psychiatric disorders, and a recent meta-analysis of its effectiveness supports such conclusions (Butler, Chapman, Forman, & Beck, 2006).

Evidence of the effectiveness of CBT in conjunction with the antidepressant fluorine in the treatment of adolescent depression is available (Treatment for Adolescents with Depression Study Team, 2004). Coming full circle now is evidence suggesting that some of the hallmark exercises from positive psychology have positive effects on preventing depression in some children and youths (Cardemil, Reivich, Beevers, Seligman, & James, 2007; Reivich et al., July 2006). Finally, Seligman, Rashid, and Parks (2006) summarized two recent studies, on what they term "positive psychotherapy" (PPT), that looked at the effects of positive psychology interventions with persons who had unipolar depression. The first showed significantly decreased depression; this improvement was maintained for longer than a year after intervention. The second, which compared PPT with "therapy as usual" and with such usual treatment plus medication, resulted in higher remission rates in the PPT group. Seligman and colleagues concluded: "Together these studies suggest that treatments for depression may usefully be supplemented by exercises that explicitly increase positive emotion, engagement and meaning" (2006, p. 774).

Recognizing the value of interventions designed to maximize happiness (broadly defined) is crucially important to our work as counselors. But another responsibility for clinicians counseling from a wellness perspective lies in helping their clients to develop the skills that permit a realistic view of their circumstances. Seligman and colleagues (2006) make a related point, noting that even though the emphasis is on using core strengths to solve problems, and using positive psychology's exercises and interventions to decrease depression, specific problems are never ignored.

## The Importance of Resilience and Optimism for Successful Communication Counseling

Another look at Box 2.2, which summarizes the characteristics of the previously described Vietnam veterans who did not have PTSD following their lengthy imprisonment, makes clear the importance of optimism and resilience in fostering mental health. This is the next topic of discussion.

For many years, under the leadership of Karen Reivich and Jane Gillham, the University of Pennsylvania has conducted workshops and classes designed to teach resilience skills. To date, eleven studies have evaluated the effectiveness of such training programs, referred to collectively as the Penn Resilience Programs (PRPs), both for parents and for children and adolescents at risk for depression across a variety of cultural settings, and for students at the University of Pennsylvania. Eight of these studies are summarized in the article by Gillham and colleagues (in press). These programs require active participation in activities that encourage and reward persons for recognizing and then changing the thinking patterns that limit their effectiveness in dealing with the exigencies of everyday life. Box 2.4 lists the basic skills needed to understand one's own explanatory style and to learn to develop more accurate thinking styles. More on explanatory style is found throughout this book.

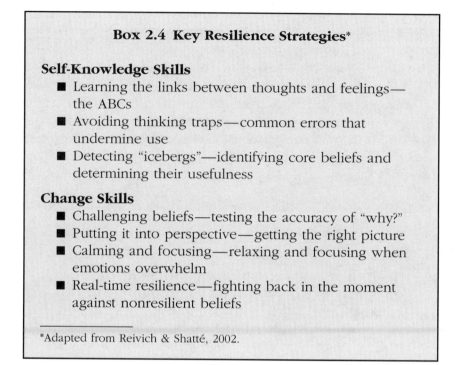

**Box 2.4 Key Resilience Strategies\***

**Self-Knowledge Skills**
- Learning the links between thoughts and feelings—the ABCs
- Avoiding thinking traps—common errors that undermine use
- Detecting "icebergs"—identifying core beliefs and determining their usefulness

**Change Skills**
- Challenging beliefs—testing the accuracy of "why?"
- Putting it into perspective—getting the right picture
- Calming and focusing—relaxing and focusing when emotions overwhelm
- Real-time resilience—fighting back in the moment against nonresilient beliefs

\*Adapted from Reivich & Shatté, 2002.

Reivich and Shatté's book *The Resilience Factor* (2002) is critical reading in this regard. Chapter 8 presents some models for workshops designed to promote resilience and wellness for individuals and families with communication disorders. Study of their book is a prerequisite for implementing such workshops. Reivich and Shatté have worked with a company called Reflective Learning (www.reflectivelearning.com) to develop online versions of their resilience programs. These programs teach the core optimism and resilience skills using interactive exercises to develop specific skills for adults, adolescents, and college students. The programs are relevant for communication counselors, with substantial applications to the populations served by SLP-As.

Of particular relevance, the most popular course on the Harvard campus, with 900 students enrolled during the 2006 winter term, was Tal Ben-Shahar's course on positive psychology, as reported on NPR (Ben-Shahar, 2006). Dr. Shahar's six tips for happiness, largely representing the range of the issues raised in this chapter, are listed in Box 2.5.

## Box 2.5 Six Tips for Happiness*

1. **Give yourself permission to be human.** When we accept emotions—such as fear, sadness, or anxiety—as natural, we are more likely to overcome them. Rejecting our emotions, positive or negative, leads to frustration and unhappiness.

2. **Happiness lies at the intersection between pleasure and meaning.** Whether at work or at home, the goal is to engage in activities that are both personally significant and enjoyable. When this is not feasible, make sure you have happiness boosters, moments throughout the week that provide you with both pleasure and meaning.

3. **Keep in mind that happiness is mostly dependent on our state of mind, not on the status or state of our bank account.** Barring extreme circumstances, our level of well-being is determined by what we choose to focus on (the full or the empty part of the glass) and by our interpretation of external events. For example, do we view failure as catastrophic, or do we see it as a learning experience?

4. **Simplify!** We are, generally, too busy, trying to squeeze in more and more activities into less and less time. Quantity influences quality, and we compromise on our happiness by trying to do too much.

5. **Remember the body-mind connection.** What we do—or don't do—with our bodies influences our minds. Regular exercise, adequate sleep, and healthy eating habits lead to both physical and mental health.

6. **Express gratitude, whenever possible.** We too often take our lives for granted. Learn to appreciate and savor the wonderful things in life, from people to food, from nature to a smile.

*From Tal Ben-Shahar's Positive Psychology class at Harvard University, 2006. Reprinted with permission from National Public Radio Archives, March 22, 2006.

## Summary

This chapter reviews the major tenets of positive psychology, particularly as they are relevant to communication counseling. The most important points are outlined, but more extensive and nuanced reading is necessary for complete understanding. A key concept is that there is great value in learning more about positive psychology, not only for clients but for clinicians and counselors as well. This is, after all, *normal*, not *abnormal*, psychology, and its benefits can certainly apply to counselors as well.

## References

American Psychiatric Association. (1994). *Diagnostic and statistical manual of mental disorders* (4th ed.). Washington, DC: Author.

Aspinwall, L. G., & Barnhart, S. M. (2000). What I do know won't hurt me: Optimism, attention to negative information, coping, and heath. In J. E. Gillham (Ed.), *The science of optimism and hope: Research essays in honor of Martin E. P. Seligman* (pp. 162–200). Philadelphia: Templeton Foundation.

Aspinwall, L. G., Richter, L., & Hoffman, R. R. (2001). Understanding how optimism "works": An examination of optimists' adaptive moderation of belief and behavior. In E. C. Chang (Ed.), *Optimism and pessimism: Theory, research, and practice* (pp. 217–238). Washington: American Psychological Association.

Aspinwall, L., & Staudinger, U. (Eds.). (2004). *A psychology of human strengths: Fundamental questions and future directions for a positive psychology*. Washington, DC: American Psychological Association.

Auto Racing: Ex-Driver Becomes a Driving Force. (2005, May 28). *New York Times*.

Beck, A. T. (1973). *The diagnosis and management of depression*. Philadelphia: University of Pennsylvania Press.

Beck, A. T., Rush, A. J., Shaw, B. F., & Emery, G. (1979). *Cognitive therapy of depression*. New York: Guilford.

Ben-Shahar, T. (2006, March 22). *Finding happiness in a Harvard classroom*. National Public Radio interview.

Butler, A. C., Chapman, J. E., Forman, E. M., & Beck, A. T. (2006). The empirical status of cognitive-behavioral therapy: A review of meta-analyses. *Clinical Psychology Review, 26*, 17–31.

Cardemil, E. V., Reivich, K. A., Beevers, C. G., Seligman, M. E. P., & James, J. (in press). The prevention of depressive symptoms in low-income minority children: Two year follow-up. *Behaviour Research and Therapy*.

Chang, E. C. (Ed). (2000). *Optimism, and pessimism: Implications for theory, research and practice*. Washington, DC: American Psychological Association.

Charney, D. S. (2005). *The psychobiology of resilience to extreme stress: Implications for the prevention and treatment of mood and anxiety disorders*. Grand Rounds presentation at Mount Sinai Hospital. *Medscape Psychiatry and Mental Health, 10*, 2. Available at www.medscape.com

Chodron, P. (2000). *When things fall apart: Heart advice for difficult times*. Boston: Shambhala.

Csikszentmihalyi, M. (1990). *Flow: The psychology of optimal experience*. New York: Harper & Row.

Csikszentmihalyi, M. (1997). *Finding flow. The psychology of engagement with everyday life*. New York: Basic Books.

Diener, E., & Seligman, M. E. P. (2002). Very happy people. *Psychological Science, 13*(1), 81–84.

Elliott, T., Kurylo, M., & Rivera, P. (2002). Positive growth following an acquired physical disability. In C. R. Snyder & S. J. Lopez (Eds.), *Handbook of positive psychology* (pp. 687–699). New York: Oxford University Press.

Fitzgerald, T., Tennen, H., Affleck, G., & Pransky, G. (1993). The relative importance of dispositional optimism and control appraisals in quality of life after coronary artery bypass surgery. *Journal of Behavioral Medicine, 16*, 25–43.

Fredrickson, B. L. (1998). What good are positive emotions? *Review of General Psychology, 2*, 300–319.

Fredrickson, B. L. (2001). The role of positive emotions in positive psychology: The broaden-and-build theory of positive emotions. *American Psychologist, 56*, 218–226.

Fredrickson, B. L., & Losada, M. (2005). Positive affect and the complex dynamics of human flourishing. *American Psychologist, 60*, 678–686.

Gilbert, D. (2006). *Stumbling on happiness*. New York: Knopf.

Gillham, J. E., Reivich, K. J., Freres, D. R., Chaplin, T. M., Shatté, A. J., Samuels, B., et al. (2007). School-based prevention of depressive symptoms: Effectiveness and specificity of the Penn Resiliency Program. *Journal of Consulting & Clinical Psychology, 75*, 313–327.

Haidt, J. (2006). *The happiness hypothesis: Finding modern truth in ancient wisdom*. New York: Basic Books.

Hollon, S. D., DeRubeis, R. J., Shelton, R. C., Amsterdam, J. D., Salomon, R. M., O'Reardon, J. P., et al. (2005). Prevention of relapse following cognitive therapy vs medications in moderate to severe depression. *Archives of General Psychiatry, 62*, 417–422.

Kabat-Zinn, J. (1994). *Wherever you go, there you are*. New York: Hyperion.

Lewinsohn, P. M., Hops, H., Roberts, R., & Seeley, J. (1993). Adolescent psychopathology: I. Prevalence and incidence of depression and other DSM-III-R disorders in high school students. *Journal of Abnormal Psychology, 102*, 110–120.

Lyon, J. (1998). *Coping with aphasia*. San Diego, CA: Singular Publishing Group.

Maier, S. F., & Seligman, M. E. P. (1976). Learned helplessness: Theory and evidence. *Journal of Experimental Psychology: General, 105*(1), 3–46.

Maruta, T., Colligan, R. C., Malinchoc, M., & Offord, K. P. (2000). Optimists vs pessimists: Survival rate among medical patients over a 30-year period. *Mayo Clinic Proceedings, 75*, 140–143.

Masten, A. (2001). Ordinary magic: Resilience processes in development. *American Psychologist, 55*, 227–238.

Peterson, C. (2006). *A primer in positive psychology*. New York: Oxford University Press.

Peterson, C., & Bossio, L. M. (1991). *Health and optimism*. New York: Free Press.

Peterson, C., Maier, S. F, & Seligman, M. E. P. (1993). *Learned helplessness: A theory for the age of personal control*. New York: Oxford University Press.

Peterson, C., & Seligman, M .E. P. (2004). *Character strengths and virtues: A classification and handbook*. New York: Oxford University Press.

Reivich, K., & Shatté, A. (2002). *The resilience factor: 7 essential skills for overcoming life's inevitable obstacles*. New York: Broadway Books.

Reivich, K. J., Gillham, J., Shatté, A., & Seligman, M. E. P. (July 2006). Penn Resiliency Project. *Executive Summary*, 1–20.

Roberts, M. K., Brown, K. J., Johnson, R. J, & Reinke, J. (2002). Positive psychology for children: Development, prevention and promotion. In C. R. Snyder & S. J. Lopez (Eds.), *Handbook of positive psychology* (pp. 663–675). New York: Oxford University Press.

Schneider, S. (2001). Realistic optimism. *American Psychologist, March*, 250–259.

Segerstrom, S. C., Taylor, S. E., Kemeny, M. E., & Fahey, J. L. (1998). Optimism is associated with mood, coping, and immune change in response to stress. *Journal of Personality and Social Psychology, 74*(6), 1646–1655.

Seligman, M. E. P. (1998). *Learned optimism*. (2nd ed.) New York: Free Press

Seligman, M. E. P. (1999). The president's address. *American Psychologist, 54*, 559–562.

Seligman, M. E. P. (2002). *Authentic happiness*. New York: Free Press.

Seligman, M. E. P. (2003). Positive clinical psychology. In L. Aspinwall & U. Staudinger (Eds.), *A psychology of human strengths: Fundamental questions and future directions for a positive psychology*. Washington, DC: American Psychological Association.

Seligman, M. E. P. (2004). *Lecture notes*. Authentic happiness coaching course.

Seligman, M. E. P. (2005). Positive psychology, positive prevention, and positive therapy. In S. R. Snyder & S. J. Lopez (Eds.) *Handbook of positive psychology*. New York: Oxford University Press.

Seligman, M.E. P., & Csikszentmihalyi, M. (2000). Positive Psychology: An Introduction. *American Psychologist, 55*, 5–14.

Seligman, M. E. P., Rashid, T., & Parks, A. (2006). Positive psychotherapy. *American Psychologist, 61*, 772–788.

Seligman, M. E. P., Reivich, K., Jaycox, L., & Gillham, J. (1995). *The optimistic child*. New York: Houghton Mifflin.

Seligman, M. E. P., Steen, T. A., Park, N., & Peterson, C. (2005). Positive psychology progress: Empirical validation of interventions. *American Psychologist, 60*(5), 410–421.

Shedler, J., Mayman, M., & Manis, M. (1993). The illusion of mental health. *American Psychologist, 48*, 1117–1131.

Snyder, C. R., & Lopez, S. J. (2005). *Handbook of positive psychology*. Oxford: Oxford University Press.

Taylor, S. E., & Brown, J. D. (1988). Illusion and well-being: A social psychological perspective on mental health. *Psychological Bulletin, 103*, 193–210.

Treatment for Adolescents with Depression Study Team. (TADS). (2004). Fluoxetine, Cognitive Behavioral Therapy and their Combination for the Treatment of Adolescents with Depression Study (TADS) Randomized Controlled Trial. *Journal of the American Medical Association*, 807–820.

Vaillant, G. E. (2002). *Aging well*. Boston: Little, Brown.

Werner, E. & Smith, R. (1982). *Vulnerable but invincible: A study of resilient children and youth*. New York: McGraw-Hill.

## Websites

www.authentichappiness.org

www.positivepsychology.org

www.reflectivehappiness.com

www.reflectivelearning.com

# Chapter 3

# GOOD COUNSELORS: KNOWLEDGE, SKILLS, CHARACTERISTICS, AND ATTITUDES

In Chapter 2, SLP-As are urged to explore their strengths and to consider how to apply them productively to communication counseling. Knowing how to deploy one's strengths is a foundation on which to build counseling skills. Nevertheless, there are other important principles on which successful communication counseling is built. The first is that practitioners of communication counseling must have an extensive knowledge base concerning the disorders with which they work. Together with the specific competencies that define a clinical knowledge base, "people skills" also are critical for successful clinical careers. Indeed, both speech pathologists and audiologists have written about the clinical relevance of "social intelligence" (whether or not it is among one's signature strengths) (Rao, 2006; Taylor, 2005). Technical counseling skills, such as active listening, affirming, and disclosing, also are crucial. This chapter briefly reviews the necessary knowledge base for communication disorders and related professional issues, identifies desirable "people skills," and describes the requisite technical counseling skills for SLP-As.

# Maintaining a Professional Knowledge Base

Competent management of speech, language, and hearing disorders depends to some significant degree on an understanding of anatomy and physiology. Counselors must understand what is normal and what specific abnormalities result in which particular disorders. Furthermore, many of the disorders and impairments we treat are caused by medical conditions that have more generalized effects and often overshadow the communication disorder itself. All clinicians must have technical, accurate, and current knowledge about the anatomy and physiology of any disorder that is the focus of their counseling. In addition, clinicians must have state-of-the-art knowledge of the clinical methods they employ, and must maintain best practices in relation to the disorders with which they work. In this context, "being knowledgeable" means integrating all such disorder-specific information into direct management of the communication problem.

In communication counseling, medical facts usually take center stage—or at least they loom in the background like the proverbial 600-pound gorilla. Many of the counseling concerns faced by parents of babies who are at risk for communication problems, or of children who have already demonstrated problems, are part of a larger medical picture. That is, although communication disorders may look to be in the foreground to us, the background of the precipitating condition invariably is at least as big, if not a bigger issue to the client. This also is true (almost without exception) of adults with late-onset disorders ranging from speech problems resulting from a laryngectomy for laryngeal cancer to language problems secondary to Alzheimer's disease. So it is appropriate for clinicians to acquire and maintain a good general knowledge base of relevant medical issues to use in counseling clients with communication disorders. What follows is a strategy for obtaining the requisite information.

One way to start is with the less personal, more general medical factors that influence counseling. Although wide individual variation is to be expected, competent counselors work with people, not with statistics or group trends. They must thoroughly understand the medical background of each communication disorder. It also is important to know the limitations of medical knowledge concerning the disease processes at hand, and to be continually alert for potential medical breakthroughs that can influence communication counseling. What follows are a few of the major issues, along with examples.

## What Is the Time Course for a Given Disorder?

Communication disorders have varying time courses that, in turn, affect clinical management. Many disorders of both children and adults are chronic to some degree and will remain so, regardless of the elegance of the clinical intervention. Helping individuals, families and caretakers to avoid pessimism and to develop a more positive outlook is both complex and difficult for problems such as raising a child with a severe hearing loss or with cerebral palsy. Help for these problems must be moored to a realistic, long-term perspective. Communication counselors are often called upon to deal with questions concerning developmental milestones that reflect (or predict) normal development, or changes in speech or language that should occur simply as a function of maturation. Parents of at-risk babies face an uncertain future. In the case of adults, related questions concern the time frame during which spontaneous changes (both positive and negative) might be expected. Answers to these questions must be individually determined and can vary markedly.

Furthermore, available guidelines concerning the time frame for spontaneous change are only approximate and often controversial. A good example is the expected duration of spontaneous recovery following a stroke. Such issues challenge the counselor's skills. Nonetheless, having some secure knowledge available, as well as some understanding of the limitations of that knowledge, is a professional responsibility of the skilled communication counselor. For example, an unfortunate and largely inadvertent byproduct of post-stroke rehabilitation is that individuals and families often develop the notion that they are in a race against time. They assume that when time spent in intensive rehabilitation is completed, no subsequent positive change will occur. Rehabilitation staff may sometimes unintentionally convey this message, and current patterns for reimbursement of services certainly reinforce it. The idea that there will be no more gains, however, is depressing and, in most cases, untrue. The communication counselor should address such time-related issues, which are revisited in Chapter 6.

Parents of children with a variety of potential developmental disabilities face parallel issues with the passage of time. When babbling fails to occur in the same time frame as that recalled for Claudia's older sister, or when the first words do not appear by 15 months, what does it mean? Is Claudia retarded? These questions worry even parents who believe their children are developing normally, but they are especially loaded for parents of children who have disabilities. Can catch-up happen? What if it doesn't? Can we meaningfully predict Claudia's future? Again, these are time-related issues that constitute fertile ground for counseling.

## What Is this Disorder's Pattern of Change?

Some neurogenic communication disorders, such as those associated with traumatic brain injury (TBI) improve over time; others, like those accompanying amyotrophic lateral sclerosis (ALS), have a pattern of progressive deterioration. Patterns of recovery or deterioration play an important role in clinical management and influence clinical decision-making by the person with the disorder, family members, the referring physician, and the communication counselor. For the type of collaborative, shared decision-making emphasized in this book, the projected pattern of recovery or deterioration often is a crucial piece of information.

Deteriorating patterns are seldom pertinent for speech, language, and hearing disorders in children, in whom the time course of development and maturation typically is positive, if sometimes slow and meandering. But exceptions do occur. For example, deterioration may occur in children whose normal development is interrupted by frequent hospitalizations for ongoing medical problems, or in apparently normally developing two-year-olds with a late-developing autism spectrum disorder (Rogers, 2004). In such cases, the counseling issues may have much longer trajectories, but parental concerns resemble those of a family in which an adult member incurs a disorder such as Alzheimer's disease.

## What Problems Accompany and Influence the Disorder?

Many speech, language, and hearing disorders are accompanied by other problems that can influence counseling, as well as direct language and speech intervention. For example, in the case of right hemisphere stroke, the effect of anosognosia and neglect on language and speech can be substantial. Depression also is common in communication disorders, and parents and partners of the affected person are at risk as well. As noted earlier, communication counselors must be particularly alert to this possibility.

Pharmacological interventions often have a profound effect on communication and such effects need to be well understood and anticipated. Communication counselors must pay particular attention to the effects of antiepileptic medications on children who are prone to seizure disorders. Some antiepileptic drugs (AEDs) also may have primary effects on communication. For example, topiramate is reputed to have negative effects on language, particularly affecting word-finding skills, in children (Kockelmann, Elger, & Helmstaedter, 2004). Adults with brain damage are especially vulnerable to antipsychotic medications, which are likely to affect cognition negatively (Maguire, 2000). For further information concerning pharmacology and communication, recommended reading includes works by Vogel, Carter, and Carter (1999), Johnson and Jacobson (1998), and Golper (1992). The communication counselor must be alert to the range of medication-associated problems. Because the medication scene is likely to change frequently, it is imperative for communication counselors to stay current.

Finally, many communication disorders are accompanied by motor, cognitive and emotional factors, and furthermore, they often occur in complex social situations. Consider, for example, the myriad problems faced by children with cerebral palsy, TBI, or autism. Communication counselors must be able to place the speech, language, or hearing disorder in its proper perspective when it comes embedded in a tangled package of problems, some directly affecting children, others directly affecting parents and thereby indirectly affecting children.

## Are Expectations Appropriate?

Communication counseling is enhanced when family, client, and clinician all have well-grounded expectations. Effective counseling depends on the clinician's awareness of probable outcomes for a given disorder. Parents, families, or individual clients need to have realistic and modulated, but nonetheless positive, expectations. For example, knowing that glioblastoma multiformae is a particularly virulent tumor tempers both how to counsel individuals and their families about the communication problem it brings and how to approach rehabilitation. The following scenario illustrates some of the considerations that may arise:

> Lily was a beautiful, buoyant 14-year-old girl who developed a fast-growing glioblastoma. Worried about her worsening anomia, Lily and her parents decided to follow her neurosurgeon's advice to consider language therapy. Both parents believed that the quality of Lily's life, however short, could be enhanced by positive, forward-looking interactive activities with a sensitive clinician. Accordingly, once-weekly therapy was undertaken for the 3 months that preceded her death. Counseling was an integral part of Lily's speech therapy.
>
> Even as Lily lost ground, she continued to smile, to worry about her appearance, and to anticipate the weekly visits and the carefully orchestrated conversations with her clinician. Her parents made the decision for intervention with a full understanding of the facts of Lily's disorder. It was part of their commitment to help her live her remaining days with hope. Another family facing the same problem, but with a different agenda and in different circumstances, could easily have made a different decision, with equal justification.

## Related Professional Competence Issues

Two additional areas of importance in a discussion of professional competence are (1) the referral process and (2) knowledge about community and Internet resources.

### Referral Issues

As noted in Chapter 1, clinicians sometimes have difficulty with the boundaries between communication counseling and counseling for accompanying problems. Some clinicians face this boundary issue with queasiness; others scurry away altogether. For ethical reasons, communication counselors must recognize when the client's problem is beyond the scope of SLP-A clinical practice. The irony is that for communication counselors, this challenge is complicated by the very nature of their skills, particularly with adult clients who have language disorders. The "talking therapies" all revolve around just that—talking. Even when the problems are beyond their expertise, communication counselors are likely to understand the language and speech used to express them. Conversely, counselors and therapists from other professions face a significant barrier when attempting to help disordered individuals who have substantial communication disorders.

Skillful counselors respect the boundaries and limitations of their counseling skills and responsibilities. They also must know how to seek information from fellow professionals (particularly psychologists or social workers) and determine if co-treatment is an option. Finally, they must have a comprehensive understanding of a given community's referral resources for persons with communication disorders and know how to use the referral process. Developing such a database takes extensive exploration and networking with relevant professionals in one's community, but, in the long run, it pays off in more efficient and appropriate referrals.

## Information about Community and Internet Resources

In additional to professional referral sources, competent counselors also know about general community resources, such as senior citizen centers, access to public transportation for people with disabilities, disorder-specific support groups, experimental clinical and research programs, and so forth. Internet resources are of growing importance, and websites are available for all of the disorders discussed in this book. Comprehensive published summaries of these rich and varied sources of information are available; see the article by Kuster (2000) as an example.

Programs that facilitate access to the Internet for people with neurogenic communication disorders and their families are becoming increasingly available (Worrall & Egan, 2000). The competent counselor knows about these resources and also about many excellent self-help books and personal accounts that can enhance counseling efforts. One of the strengths of Internet resources, of course, is that they are in a state of almost constant flux, with almost constant updating. This is exciting, to be sure, but keeping up is crucial and often frustrating.

## Competent Counselors: Personal Characteristics

In his text on clinical skills in speech-language pathology, Goldberg (1997) notes that lists of characteristics suffer from their lack of operational definitions. Nonetheless, some of these word pictures set the tone of what it means to be an effective clinician. Rogers' (1965) notion of *unconditional positive regard* for one's clients has always been a foundation, if not a mantra, for my own clinical practice, however lacking in operationalism it may be. Satir's (1967) compilation of desirable characteristics for clinicians who provide conjoint family therapy has a special resonance for communication counseling. The most relevant characteristics are listed in Box 3.1.

The issue of personal characteristics of effective communication counselors can be approached in a number of ways. Because self-knowledge is such a fundamental characteristic of good coun-

---

**Box 3.1 Some Characteristics of Successful Clinicians***

- Reveal yourself clearly to others.
- Be in touch with your feelings and capabilities.
- Regard each person as unique.
- Differences are learning experiences, not threats or signals for conflict.
- Understand clients for who they are, not how you wish them to be.
- Understand that clients are responsible for their own behaviors.

---

*Adapted from Satir, V. (1967). *Conjoint family therapy* (rev. ed.). Palo Alto, CA: Science and Behavior Books.

selors, looking at one's own strengths is a good place to begin, as has already been suggested. This section presents some basic questions about personal qualities that appear to be central to effective counseling. The questions and their elaborations provided are neither overwhelming nor comprehensive; they simply illustrate some personal characteristics that help people to be good counselors. Evaluate yourself in relation to them, and study the rationales for each characteristic.

## Are You a Good Listener?

Most counseling texts stress the importance of being a good listener. But what are the qualities of a "good listener"? Good listeners listen actively and non-judgmentally. My friend Elisabet Sahtouris has remarked that good listening is "willingness to have one's mind changed by what one hears" (personal communication, Sahtouris, 2006). I certainly concur.

Good listeners are alert not only to what is being said but to what underlies the comments, what motivates them, and what meanings they have for the speaker. Theodore Reik (1948) referred to this process of listening both to surface and latent content of a message as "listening with the third ear." It is true that some people are born listeners, but listening skills also are teachable and learnable. Finally, good listeners know that listening is active. So now if you hear someone saying, "I didn't do anything—I just listened," you will recognize the inherent contradiction: The concept of "just listening" cannot coexist with the active process required. Some listening exercises are presented in Box 3.2.

## Are You an Active Constructive Responder?

Gable, Reis, Impett, and Asher (2004) provide an excellent model for maximally effective responding to what one has been listening to. Although their work centered on relationships among partners and on responses to positive events, their findings have strong implications for parenting, for counseling, and for negative events as well.

## Box 3.2 Two Exercises in Listening

### Exercise 1: Listening for surface and latent content

**A.** Listening requires active attending to what is being said and then responding appropriately. Listening involves being aware that content can be transmitted at two levels—that is, the manifest and the latent. Both must be listened for. Finally, listening also involves being aware of both nonverbal and verbal behavior and searching for mismatches and congruities between them. Putting yourself on the sending end of this process, list six ways in which a person might communicate the following message: "I don't want to talk about this any more."

**B.** For each of the following messages, identify one or more possible beneath-the-surface meanings:

■ Ellen comments, "Oh, you like horror movies—that's interesting," while simultaneously swiveling her body away from and breaking eye contact with Rob, her conversational partner.

■ George comments, "It's really hard to listen to Grandma because she talks constantly."

■ Nora says, "You look great in that dress. I wish I also could wear clothes designed for younger women."

### Exercise 2: Latent Message and Locus of Responsibility

In each of the following requests for repair, what is the latent message? Where does the speaker place responsibility? Why does it matter?

■ "I wish you would speak a bit louder."

■ "I'm afraid this is not one of my good listening days. I missed that."

■ "Could you go over that again?"

■ "Let's see if I got that."

■ "It would be much easier for me if you spoke slowly and clearly."

The following hypothetical example concerns an 11-year-old client with diagnosed speech-language impairment (SLI):

> Mackenzie tells you that her poster concerning safety issues for children won the school's top award. According to Gable and associates (2004), responses to such events can take one of four possible forms:
>
> - **Active constructive responding:** "That's great! I bet you'll be doing more good art after this."
> - **Active destructive responding:** "Don't get too carried away. Now they'll expect you to enter all the contests."
> - **Passive constructive responding:** "That's swell."
> - **Passive destructive responding** (a response that signals your lack of interest in or regard for the person): "I didn't know you could draw."

Gable and colleagues' (2004) data on response patterns of married couples indicate that active constructive responses predominate in good marriages. When any of the other response types predominates, less satisfying marriages are the result. The use of active constructive responding has much bigger implications, however. There is no doubt that active constructive responding is not always appropriate (for example, if Mackenzie tells you that her cat has been hit by a car). Gable and associates (2004) suggest that for strong effects, active constructive responses need to occur along with other responses, such as passive constructive, passive negative and active negative responses in a ratio greater than 3:1.

> How do the four response types stack up for negative events?
>
> Mackenzie reports her bitter disappointment over not winning the contest:
>
> - Active constructive responding: "I am so sorry to hear that. It must feel really awful, especially since you are such a good artist. But we have to figure out how to do better next time."
> - Active destructive responding: "I guess Jill is just a better artist than you are."
> - Passive constructive responding: "You are feeling pretty bad."
> - Passive destructive responding: "It was just a school contest, after all."

Many of us have been inculcated with the notion that neutral, reflective, nondirective responding is preferred in clinical interaction. In the foregoing scheme, this type of responding is passive constructive. Although this kind of response may be meaningful in psychotherapeutic interactions, the active constructive approach often seems a better fit with the counseling roles and responsibilities of SLP-As. Box 3.3 provides some opportunities to explore all four types of responding, for both positive and negative reports.

---

### Box 3.3 Exercise: Clinical Response Types

For each of the following clinical scenarios, provide an active-constructive, an active destructive, a passive-constructive, and a passive-destructive response to both the positive and the negative comments.

The client is Sybil, a young woman with mild TBI. She reports:
- "I think I got the part-time job I applied for."
- "I don't think I got that part-time job."

The client is Ned, the father of 8-year-old Teddy, who stutters. He comments:
- "Teddy got picked to start the Little League game on Saturday."
- "Teddy wasn't selected to start the Little League game on Saturday."

The client is Elise, spouse of Wilton, who has chronic dysphagia. She says:
- "We had two couples over for dinner, and it was a disaster."
- "We had two couples over for dinner, and it went just fine."

The client is Geoff, who has severe presbyacusis. He says:
- "The new hearing aids work just fine. I heard the sermon at church, for a change."
- "The new hearing aids are as bad as the old ones. I still can't hear the sermon."

## Are You a Good Communicator?

It is not necessary, and probably not desirable, for counselor-clinicians to aspire to be eloquent. Rather, being a good communicator in this context refers to the ability to reach clients or family members on their terms and at their level of understanding, and to communicate with body language as diverse as getting down on the floor with a small child or holding the hand of a grieving spouse. Box 3.4 provides some practice exercises for translating professional jargon to families and patients.

## Can You Listen Comfortably to People Who Have Trouble Talking?

The very nature of communication disorders makes listening even more basic for SLP-As than it is for counselors in other disciplines, primarily because reduced intelligibility often presents an additional challenge. How do you handle situations in which you might fail to

---

**Box 3.4**
**Exercise: Translating Professional Jargon**

Put the following statements into normal English:

"In addition to his difficulty with auditory comprehension, Mr. J seems to me to have a severe limb apraxia."

"Johnny's sensorimotor skills seem to lag behind his cognitive abilities."

"We are going to have to be very careful about the consistency of Mrs. S's oral intake, in order to avoid having her aspirate."

"I really think that the low intensity of Mr. T's speech contributes disproportionately to his lack of intelligibility."

"It is not uncommon for children who have phonological processing disorders to become dyslexic as they mature."

understand what is being said to you, regardless of how actively and patiently you are listening? How easy is it for you to admit that you don't understand? How comfortable can you make the speaker whose speech intelligibility is an issue?

Because intelligibility can be a challenging problem, one interesting way to practice listening skills is by eavesdropping on fellow clinicians and their clients and second-guessing their communication problems and solutions. Another is to develop a repertoire of graceful ways to admit lack of understanding in advance and use them when needed. "Faking it" is truly not an option. Almost all of us have tried it at one point or another; however, once caught by your client, you probably will not want to try it again. It is costly in terms of rapport, and your own embarrassment takes a toll too. Here is an example:

> **Client:** (*Unintelligible sentence*)
>
> **Clinician:** (*Hoping to move on*) "Sure, that sounds like a good idea."
>
> **Client:** (*Dysarthrically*) "What did I just say?" (Incidentally, the client's latent message is "Gotcha!")

Similar client interactions, with resulting professional embarrassment, have no doubt ensnared every clinician at least once. Box 3.5 provides some practice on how to handle such situations.

---

**Box 3.5**
**Exercise: Talking to Clients Who Are**
**Difficult to Understand**

You are talking with your client Bunny, a person of the opposite sex who has moderate executive system dysfunction and severe dysarthria following a TBI. Bunny asks you a question that you do not understand, but you say "yes" anyway. Bunny then says (intelligibly): "What did I ask you?" What do you say?

## Can You Listen to Emotions?

Communication problems inevitably have emotional consequences, often including crying and sadness, frequently realized in tears. In addition, some disorders (e.g., strokes) may bring inadvertent crying or laughing as a result of brainstem involvement. The one inviolate rule is that crying should be acknowledged.

Clinical viewpoints vary on the form of such acknowledgment. As borne out in my own clinical experience, helpful and authentic responses may include gently taking a hand, offering a tissue, and encouraging verbal expression of the emotion behind the tears. Such behavior is in fact part of the listening process, and crying is to be honored as something the client is willing to share. Regardless of how the individual SLP-A decides to deal with crying, all counselors should plan an appropriate response for use in clinical practice. The following scenario illustrates possible adverse consequences of lack of such a plan:

> A student clinician was summarizing the results of a long afternoon of exhaustive testing for a client with aphasia, who probably was confronting the magnitude of his language problem for the first time, and who also was fatigued from his efforts in the testing process. His wife was present. As the clinician was listing his problems and telling him about the long therapy road ahead, he burst into tears. The student clinician continued her report matter-of-factly, ignoring both the man's tears and his wife's concern. At the end of her litany she asked, "Are there any questions?" When none were forthcoming, she stood, they stood, and all left the room.
>
> Her clinical supervisor greeted them in the hall and attempted to ameliorate the situation. Later, when the supervisor asked the student why she had ignored the emotional scene, the student replied, "I didn't know what to do. In the American culture, men are not supposed to cry, and I decided that the best way to help him was to pretend I didn't notice!"

Besides tears, clinicians also have to listen to overtly negative emotions. Communication counseling can involve anger, frustration, and anxiety. Some of us can handle these emotions with equanimity;

for others, they are very threatening. Of note, the anger, the frustration, and the anxiety are almost without exception never about *you*. It's more likely that they find their way to you because something else altogether has triggered a client's negativity and you were close by. Alternatively (and ironically), you may have engendered enough trust to permit the client to feel safe about sharing negative things with you. When the negative emotions fly, take a deep breath while trying to remember that they are not about you. Box 3.6 presents some exercises for you to use to explore these issues on your own.

---

**Box 3.6**
**Exercise: Fielding Negative Emotions**

For each of the following client comments projecting discomfort or distress, provide a helpful and appropriate response.

"It makes me wonder about the genes on my wife Linda's side of the fence. I know for certain that nothing like this has ever happened in *my* family before."

"If you're gonna be my therapist, you'd better get to know me a bit. I smoke, and I don't want to hear about it. I also don't want you to be on my case for swearing. You can just forget that little goody-two-shoes routine if you work with me, honey."

"You're just like all the rest! Nobody around here tells me anything that is helpful! I am sooooo frustrated about what's happening! I don't even know what the plans are for next week! Does every parent with a TBI kid get such treatment, or am I special?"

"Is this for real, or what? The doctor says he's doing fine. You say he can't eat normal food. What am I supposed to do?"

"Okay, I'm taking her home tomorrow, and I don't have a clue about how this is all going to work. Don't any of you people worry about that?"

"Nobody ever prepared me for this! Who do they think I am—Einstein?"

---

## Can You Listen to Ideas That Conflict with Your Values?

In clinical practice, communication counselors are likely to encounter people whose values and attitudes differ markedly from their own. Value differences can arise in relation to almost any controversial issue, from religious practices to sexual orientation. Attempting to change people's values, even when they are personally repugnant to you, is absolutely beyond the scope of clinical practice.

Values also affect issues that seem less controversial, such as the importance of speech therapy or hearing aids. Our professional culture views them as necessary in many cases, and probably even imperative. Clients may see things differently. How do value differences affect our ability to make and maintain clinically useful contact? Satir's earlier-quoted notion of accepting "who they are" rather than "how we might wish them to be" has important implications for communication counseling.

Another way to approach differences in values is to develop the ability to take another's perspective. The effectiveness of the counseling process often depends on being able to see things as the other sees them. Empathy, for example, is rooted in the ability to shift perspective. Many things we ask clients to do clinically may seem opaque to them, or not clearly related to improving speech, language, hearing, or swallowing. Seeing our tactics through another person's eyes increases our insight into how we may present information.

## Are You Sensitive to Cultural Differences?

All therapeutic endeavors occur in cultural contexts. Thus, cultural factors demand awareness and sensitivity in our roles as clinicians and counselors. When a clinician fails to understand and accept the cultural values of a particular client and family and, as a result, fails to place various clinical activities within the mores and beliefs of that culture, clinical intervention will be unsuccessful. This is true even when all of the work is done with sincere good will and honesty.[1]

---

[1] For a poignant and instructive example, read Fadiman's remarkable book *The Spirit Catches You and You Fall Down* (1997), an exploration of a clash of American medical values and those of a family of the Hmong culture.

Clinicians must take the steps necessary to develop cultural sensitivity that is intrinsic to their success. Some texts that are particularly relevant to multicultural concerns in communication counseling are those by Payne (1997), Goldberg (1997), Wallace (1993), and Battle (2003). A comprehensive bibliography is available at the American Speech-Language-Hearing Association (ASHA) website (http://www. asha.org) through the link entitled "General issues and multicultural populations."

Understanding a client's culture is critical to successful counseling. Effective counselors learn about the cultural backgrounds of the persons with whom they work, a task that becomes increasingly daunting as society becomes more culturally diverse. At a minimum, effective counselors must respect and accept cultural differences. Value and culture issues are explored in Box 3.7.

### Are You Optimistic and Positive?

Many disorders that fall within the scope of practice for SLP-As appear to be bleak, and many deal with tragedy. To be effective counselors, SLP-As must remain realistically optimistic and actively seek the positive. Reality, as Schneider points out, is fuzzy, and so is knowledge (Schneider, 2001).[2] Because communication disorders are complex in nature, clinicians and counselors who are technically skilled in working with affected persons and their families also must be affirming and upbeat. This is important not only for helping families and clients to discover ways to "broaden and build," as discussed in Chapter 2, but because clinicians need these qualities to avoid burnout. Clinicians who remain enthusiastic and positive, who are able to look on the bright side, and who are fascinated by complex problems can make a gift of their optimism to the persons with whom they work.

This quality of personal optimism should not be confused with being a "Pollyanna person"—someone who is consistently positive or forcedly cheerful even in circumstances in which such an outlook is unrealistic and therefore inappropriate. Late on a Friday afternoon, I once heard a student clinician say to a client on a respirator in an intensive care unit: "Have a great weekend." This is not recommended.

---

[2] For a thorough explanation of the complex nature of tricks that our eyes and brains play on us in this regard, see Gilbert's *Stumbling Toward Happiness* (2006).

**Box 3.7**
**Exercise: When Cultures and Values Clash**

1. Answer the questions for the following scenarios involving a clash of cultures or values.

   ■ A person states: "I am not comfortable with people who are not forthright enough to look me in the eye." Suggest a clinical/cultural encounter that might present problems for this person. If the person is the counselor, how might this expressed attitude affect a clinical interaction? If the person is a client who is the mother of a child with cerebral palsy, what are some possible effects?

   ■ An 85-year-old woman who has just had her third stroke tells you, "Go away! Leave me alone! I don't want speech therapy!" You know that her speech and language are impaired. In addition, you suspect she probably has multiple-infarct dementia and may not be thinking clearly, and that you could definitely be of help. What are some value differences that may be reflected in her comments?

2. Make a list of five personal values that you hold. For each value, name some individuals or groups of individuals whose corresponding values may differ. For example, a personal value may be stated as follows: "I believe that Western-style speech-language intervention is useful in adult neurogenic communication disorders." By contrast, some Native Americans may believe that individuals who have incurred strokes have been blessed in some special way.

## Do You Have a Good Sense of Humor?

To many clinicians, emphasizing a sense of humor may seem misplaced. Yet a working ability to see the light side, as well as the bright side, is a vital attribute of the successful counselor. Norman Cousins (1991) noted that laughter was an essential part of his recovery from a life-threatening disease. Simmons-Mackie's delicious bow to humor in aphasia therapy (2004) should be mandatory reading for all clinicians. People who can appreciate humor or even laugh at themselves probably cope better with these often messy communication disorders than persons who are more somber. Of course, many people (with and without communication disorders) are dour and humorless. However, if their clinicians and counselors have the ability to see the funny side of life, it can help to balance their own perspectives, decrease their burnout, and enliven the experiences of those with whom they work.

## Are You Flexible?

The challenging (and changing) nature of communication disorders requires those clinicians who counsel affected persons and their families to be adaptable and flexible enough to change approaches and goals in the face of new data, whether it is of a general nature, or specific to a particular person. Because of the fluid state of current health care delivery, the ability to operate effectively within the system also demands flexibility.

## Can You See Beyond the Obvious?

It is important for the clinician-counselor to be able to see beyond the obvious—to recognize more subtle psychosocial factors that may affect the counseling process—and to address any relevant problems as appropriate. Difficulties within the client's family relationships or stresses in dealing with the communication disorder may impede clinical progress, as in the following example:

> It's not hard to deduce that Tucker probably is going to have a pretty rough day in speech therapy, because he and his mother arrive late and apparently frazzled for today's session with you. In addition, his mother forgot to bring his implant device along. Moreover, Tucker's mother asks you the same questions every week and shows virtually no follow-through on any of the plans you have sent home with her, or the advice you have given her.

What do the lateness, the forgetfulness, the repetitive questioning, and the lack of follow-through all mean? Are they related? Putting two and two together, you decide that they are: They say "anxious mom"—and an anxious mom can be a real stumbling block to Tucker's success. Her anxiety must be acknowledged and dealt with if Tucker is to thrive.

## Do You Know Yourself? Do You Like Yourself?

Self-respect, self-esteem, and self-knowledge have always been core issues for counselors in any area of counseling. Communication counseling is no different. Self-examination is an ongoing but rewarding process whereby self-acceptance can be achieved. Many approaches to the development of self-acceptance, ranging from formal psychotherapy to disciplined meditation, are recognized. Whichever approach is used, spending time periodically examining one's own life leads to increasing self-acceptance, an important attribute of the successful counselor.

Self-knowledge can be developed in various ways. To begin, communication counselors can look to their own clinical work to uncover clues in this regard. It is helpful to become aware of issues such as the following: "Why am I pleased when this client cancels a session?" "Where does my anger with this client come from?" "Why does a session with this family make me happy?" or "Why do I leave my session with this client feeling sad?" Self-examination on this basis often reveals underlying feelings that, when attended to properly, can clarify some issues regarding not only clients but also ourselves.

## Do You Like Challenges?

The management of many communication and swallowing disorders is, without doubt, challenging. Such disorders are baffling in their inconsistency and variability. Some entail dealing with end-of-life issues. Communication disorders occur across a spectrum of complex social contexts. They must be treated with little time and even less money, and often in less than ideal environments. For the person who is threatened, rather than energized by challenges, this field may not be suitable.

Some years ago, I asked students in a counseling class to write a brief description of their ideal clients. The next week they each in turn described this mythical person. As the composite morphed in my head, I became quite discouraged. Their ideal client was Mythical Mary Sue, a sweet little eight-year-old girl, dressed to perfection (in pink). Mary Sue did just what the clinician asked her to do, and why not? She had a perfect home life, with parents who did every clinic assignment with their perfectly cooperative and uncomplaining daughter, and she became perfectly cured of her slight phonological problem by the end of the scheduled treatment plan. Halfway through the presentations, I stopped them. "Do you mean this?" I shouted as I summarized perfect little Mythical Mary Sue. "Where's the fun? Where's the challenge? Give little Mary Sue a break! She's so perfect she'll get to be Miss America even if she lisps!"

The class cracked up but got the point. Fortunately, Mary Sue seldom shows up on real clinical caseloads, because challenge, not boredom, is much more likely to energize the effective clinician-counselor. Box 3.8 contains a related exercise to help you learn about yourself as a clinician.

## Attitudes

In his famous book *Man's Search for Meaning* (1989), Victor Frankl describes certain prisoners in concentration camps who

---

**Box 3.8**
**Exercise: Personal Attitudes and Client Characteristics:**
**The Ideal versus the "Nightmare" Client**

1. Write a paragraph or two describing your ideal client. What makes him or her so appealing to you?
2. Now do the opposite: Describe your nightmare client. What characteristics give you problems? Are they yours or the client's?

spent their days taking care of others in whatever ways they could. He points out:

> They may have been few in number, but they offer sufficient proof that everything can be taken from a man but one thing: The last of his freedoms—to choose one's attitude in any given set of circumstances, to choose one's own way. (Frankl, 1989, p. 104)

How we respond to challenge leads directly to a discussion of attitudes. Counselors' attitudes about their roles help to determine the success of their counseling. The following review of attitudes in clinical practice[3] borrows heavily from Webster's (1977) discussion of appropriate attitudes for counselors who work with families of handicapped children.

Particularly critical for communication counselors are the following factors: how one views oneself in relationship to others, how one perceives and handles issues in authority, and, finally, what attitudes one has about the issue of control. Each of these factors is discussed next.

## Relationships with Others

Webster (1977) reminds her readers of Martin Buber's (1958) notion of the "I-Thou and "I-It" dichotomies. When one person approaches another as Thou in a relationship, the other person is respected or even revered. In I-It relationships, the other person is objectified— treated as a subject for analysis. I-It relationships are important for many aspects of interpersonal relationships. For example, it is important to remember and respect others' preferences about many things and to categorize and know facts about others to whom one is close.

But in the I-Thou relationship, the respect (and value) one holds for others is holistic. It is based not on attributes or facts but on an individual's very personhood. Furthermore, I-Thou relationships preclude analysis and dissection and insist on acceptance.

---

[3]Development of the ideas that follow has been greatly influenced by my mentors, Elizabeth Webster and Louise Ward.

In relation to counseling, the I-Thou and the I-It dichotomies permit consideration of questions such as the following: "Is the information I have to offer of greater value to me than the person to whom I offer it?" "Do I see the persons I counsel as objects to be directed for their own good?" "Do I work with a disorder or with a person?"

A significant example concerns how a clinician chooses to address a client. Many older clients, for example, come from various cultures and traditions mandating that others be given permission before familiarity can be assumed. Yet it is increasingly and annoyingly common for clinicians, hospital personnel, and other health professionals to assume that first names are perfectly acceptable forms of address. (This may be exceptionally galling when the clinician or staff member is substantially younger than the client addressed.)

This issue is directly related to the I-Thou, I-It dichotomy and its effects on human interaction. It is a simple matter to ask clients how they prefer to be addressed. Clinician-counselors should never make an assumption concerning form of address; rather, they should simply ask what their clients wish to be called. This is an effective way to honor the I-Thou aspect of a clinical interaction and should be practiced by all clinicians and counselors.

### Authority and Locus of Control

The growing voice of the disability movement (e.g., Jordan & Kaiser, 1996) is influencing much of our clinical and counseling work in general. In Chapter 1, the issue of "Who is the expert?" was raised. That notion is revisited here, along with the value of collaborative models, in which individuals, families, and clinicians contribute to shared decision-making and treatment planning. Key issues relate to the nature and distribution of authority and the locus of counseling control.

One useful way to examine locus of control factors is for skilled counselors to look at themselves in relation to Fromm's (1947) description of "rational vs. irrational authority." In Fromm's view, rational authority stems from equality of the so-called authority (in this case, the counselor) and the person with whom this authority is working. Rational authority is related to competence, but authority status is earned, and others must confer it. It is temporary and dependent on changing information and new data, and the authority of others sometimes overrides it. Rational authority-type people admit their mistakes, are not easily threatened, change their minds when new information is presented, and continually seek to improve what they are doing. They treat others as "Thou" rather than "It." Irrational authority-type people, of course, hold different beliefs. They prefer having power over others, have trouble with criticism, admit mistakes slowly, and assume, rather than earn, their authority. Irrational authority types treat others as "It."

Few would like to think of themselves as irrational authority types, but a key feature of rational authority concerns the equality of the counselor and the counseled. Although the counselor has the expertise in the disorder and techniques for its management, the individual and family are specialists and experts in knowledge about themselves. The expertise of counselors lies both in the extent of their general knowledge and in the breadth of their experience with individuals who share certain problems and conditions.

On the other hand, the expertise of individuals and their families resides in the depth of their experience of the disorder and how it manifests for them. That is, they are experts on how a disorder is lived with every day, as well as on what it is like to have the disorder. Hence, a consideration of attitudes concerning locus of counseling control progresses naturally from that of I-Thou relationships and rational authority.

It is probably a good idea for clinicians to omit their professional titles when introducing themselves to a client or a family. Fromm's concept of rational authority cautions against it. In my own clinical practice, introducing myself by saying "I'm Audrey Holland," rather than "I'm Dr. Holland" (or, worse, "My name is Dr. Holland"), has averted subsequent wrangling about authority and how I am perceived. It also permits me the freedom to be myself, and to practice my clinical skills in a personally satisfying way without relying on the authority implicit in a title.

The successful communication counselor recognizes the collaborative partnership of clinician, affected person, and family and its dependence on the clinician's attitudes about control in relationship to authority. When clinicians believe that they are the authorities, others involved then become nonspecialists or novices. Webster (1977) notes:

> Counselors will get along better with parents (and we add, individuals and families) when they understand that whenever one counselor meets with one parent (or one individual with a neurogenic communication disorder, or with his or her family), there are two (or more) specialists involved (p. 67).

Webster (1977) goes on to say that perhaps counselors should consider the following question: To what extent do I believe I can solve this problem? She suggests that communication counselors who feel responsible for taking the lead in solving problems are likely to provide copious amounts of advice and to feel successful only when that advice is acted upon. A better alternative involves respecting clients and their families as capable of managing their own lives, clarifying those aspects that need changing, and encouraging clients to carry out their own solutions. Thus, a good counselor should be a participant in the counseling process, not its director.

## Technical Skills

What are the basic skills of a good counselor? Numerous authorities list many different skills. Recall from Chapter 1 that Webster and Newhoff (1981) included the importance of *listening* to what others wanted to share, to clarify ideas, attitudes, emotions, beliefs, and to provide information and options for change. As listed in Box 1.1, the essential components of counseling are *understanding*, *explaining*, *advising*, and *translating* into action. Notice that these basic skills are presented as verbs They involve active or intentional processes and in fact constitute the dynamics of the counseling process. By contrast, clinician characteristics are nouns; they are static qualities that provide a background against which the active counseling skills operate.

Box 3.9 illustrates the importance of definitive action (as represented by verb forms) in the counseling process.

Notice that the skills in the first column are "quieter" than those in the second column. That is, their functions are predomi-

---

**Box 3.9  Counseling Skills: Quiet Skills and Loud Skills**

| "Quiet" Skills | "Loud" Skills |
|---|---|
| Listening and understanding | Informing and explaining |
| Empathizing | Teaching |
| Clarifying, reflecting | Advising |
| Disclosing | Planning |
| Affirming | |

---

nantly supportive in nature, whereas those in the second column—the "louder" skills—are more oriented to change and growth. Both types seem to be necessary for competent counseling, and in actual use, their boundaries frequently are blurred.

# The "Quiet" Skills

## Listening and Understanding

Listening has already been discussed. Of importance, however, *active listening* involves more than just ears. It is signaled by posture, good eye contact (at least in Western cultures), nonverbal behaviors such as head-nodding, judicious pausing, and avoiding interruption and overlaps. Indeed, use of body language to look like an attentive listener is a very important part of the listening process. Everyone has experienced instances in which someone asks (usually impatiently), "Are you listening?" That question usually is triggered not by any evidence of ear malfunction but by what the rest of the body is doing. Although listening is not synonymous with understanding, it certainly is the main requirement.

Clinicians must recognize the importance of getting beyond the words and the syntax not only when we teach language, but when we counsel. *Understanding* clearly is decoding and comprehending, but it also connotes empathy. For example, people may listen to and comprehend what a certain politician says, but they certainly do not empathize and thus do not truly understand the message behind the politician's comments (they cannot know the specific aspect of personal background or experience, for example, that led to a particular public decision or stated belief). Counselors must listen with the "third ear," as noted earlier, and in fact attend with something like the Buddhist concept of the *third eye* as well. A problem with understanding is that counselors sometimes presume to understand when in fact they may not. It is crucial to understand in order to help. Thus, many of the important counseling skills are simply ways to validate and clarify our understanding.

How do we become better, more understanding listeners? Here are some suggestions:

- Practice *full body listening*. Incorporate the culturally relevant nonverbal behaviors into listening. For a majority of persons in today's society, these behaviors include the following: leaning forward, using appropriate eye contact, nodding in agreement occasionally, and so on—in effect, *looking* like a listener.
- Ignore distractions to the listening process.
- Don't fidget.
- Try to listen with the "third eye" and "third ear." Listen for disconnect versus consistency between what is being said and the underlying message. Try to empathize.
- For clients whose intelligibility is impaired, help them to buttress their speech with writing, gestures, and other means.
- Use other counseling skills to confirm understanding.

## Empathizing

In advising health care workers how to avoid burnout, Papadatou (1997) suggests that they try to maintain an attitude of "detached concern." This attitude is almost a polar opposite of empathy, and it is difficult for me to discern how a committed communication counselor can counsel while maintaining detached concern. Many self-help books have been written on how to become more empathic. In a way, the abundance of such books is scary: If this is truly a market-driven economy, then there must be many people who feel they lack empathy. Some writers use the terms "empathy" and "compassion" as synonymous. "Sympathy" also is sometimes included, but it appears connotatively to lie closer to "pity," which seems a less desirable quality in interactions with clients. A more useful and appropriate term is "compassion," particularly in relation to counseling, because it implies a desire to be of service to others. Eric J. Cassell, a physician, described his compassion as follows:

> As I hear my patient recount the story of his illness and all its pain and sadness and see the sickness speaking from his features, my compassion is aroused. I become connected to the patient; we have begun to fuse. I am no longer in an ordinary social interaction where the "distance" between the participants is maintained and where attempts to get closer than the particular culture allows may be perceived as a broach of social convention.
>
> When that happens, I begin to listen, look, and intuit with greater intensity, and more information flows toward me. If I make myself conscious of what is happening, I can begin to feel the patient's emotions, and even my hand palpating the abdomen appears to receive more information than it otherwise would. (From Handbook of Positive Psychology C. Snyder & S. Lopez, (Editors).2005 by Oxford University Press. Reprinted with permission. p. 443)

Even without the palpating hand, Cassell's remarks serve as a model of the compassion, or empathy, that communication counselors ideally strive for. Cassell further notes that compassion is gleaned primarily through years of experience. However, the first step in achieving compassion, or empathy, comes from growing closer to what others are going through.

Experiences in our daily lives can offer empathy lessons. For example, how do you feel when you are too sick to engage in your normal life, or have to miss long-anticipated events? Or when a physician examines you with "detached concern"? Or when people give advice starting with something like "You know what you should do?" Compare these feelings with those experienced when another person communicates a sense of direct and total concern for your difficulties. Brief trips to the empathy bank do not have to wait solely on time and experience. Rather, empathy sometimes can be learned from example. Consider the examples provided by the citizens of Lake Providence discussed in Chapter 2, or the national grieving for the bombing victims that followed the 9/11 attacks.

A final note of caution: Empathy moves us along toward a feeling of walking in someone else's shoes, but it is not truly walking in them. Even when you have had an eerily parallel experience to one you are hearing about, resist the urge to say, "I know just how you feel!" In fact, no one can ever know just how another person feels. Empathy still stops short of being in another's skin. You can only know just how *you* feel.

## Clarifying and Reflecting

*Clarifying* is a two-way process, particularly in counseling clients who have communication disorders. That is, although clarifying originally was meant to cover a group of techniques whereby a counselor helps a person to understand better or to give more precise words to their own ideas and feelings, it also covers ways of making sure that the counselor actually comprehends what the speaker is saying. In both cases, the technique involves careful questioning and restatement. Some clarifying phrases intended to help clients gain self-understanding are "I think I hear you say that . . . " (and its variants) and "Let me see if I understand: Is this an example?" An especially useful clarifier is the direct request "Help me to understand."

The same kinds of clarifications can be used when it is the counselor-clinician's understanding that is of concern. One trick is to shift responsibility for communication failure from the speaker to the counselor. For example, "I'm having a bad listening day" is always useful, or "I'm missing something here . . . can you tell me again?" Compare "You probably should speak more slowly, since it's not getting through to me," or even "You need to tell me that again." Both of these place the burden of communication on the client and may inhibit his or her openness in communicating.

*Reflecting* usually is a direct application of a Rogerian nondirective therapy technique (Rogers, 1965). Reflecting refers to a strategy whereby the clinician states back to the client, or restates the underlying (latent) content of, the client's messages. It is not an exact replication of the message. For example, a man with significantly impaired speech following a stroke may state: "I am really angry at the way the health care system is jerking me around!" This could be restated as "You're feeling used by the folks down at BCD," rather than as "You are feeling really angry." The goal of reflection is to move this client forward in his ability to see his situation with increased clarity. Thus, the first response signals encouragement to be more specific about the "jerking around." The second, overly simple restatement is not nearly so likely to elicit any client response beyond "Yes, I am"—or may even precipitate "That's what I just said!" from an angry and frustrated client.

## Disclosing

*Disclosing* is the straightforward act of sharing a bit of oneself with a client. It also entails limiting disclosure to relevant issues, not sharing one's life story with a client. The goal of disclosure is similar to that of clarifying and reflecting—that is, to help the client move along with increased insight into his or her behavior. Statements such as "When my mother was sick, I felt helpless, too," for example, are appropriate forms of disclosure. So are comments that help the client to understand that you have had pertinent experiences, such as "My grandmother had Parkinson's disease, too." This kind of disclosing helps to build empathy.

Clinicians often are warned of the dangers of bringing too much of themselves into clinical interactions, and disclosing is a practice to be followed cautiously. It is a fine line to walk, but an important one. Sharing is what conversation is all about, and SLP-As, especially, recognize the importance of conversation in communication. For example, the clinician may choose to work on a topic in an aphasia conversation group such as "my most embarrassing moment." Which of the following approaches would be more likely to get the group involved?

> **Approach 1:** The clinician announces at the beginning of the session: "Today we are going to discuss our most embarrassing moments. George, think for a minute, and tell us about yours."

> **Approach 2:** "Wait till you hear what happened to me this morning when I was coming into the clinic. I think this was my most embarrassing experience ever!"

Approach 1 probably will result in silence—who would want to take a chance at such self-exposure? Approach 2 differs fundamentally: The group leader has already taken the chance, and the resulting talk is likely to be a variant on "Can you top this?" (and fun, to boot).

## Affirming

*Affirming* is the easiest of the quiet skills. Indeed, much of it is itself quiet. Affirming means communicating what Rogers calls "unconditional positive regard" (Rogers, 1992). According to this notion, the counselor is on the client's side, is there to help, and is there to understand. It is as important for clients as it is for counselors to recognize and celebrate their own strengths if they are to flourish. Affirming also can be verbal, and much of it should be, particularly if direct clinical work focuses on modifying impairment.

The *counseling moments* in subsequent chapters can serve as occasions to practice many of the quiet skills just outlined. Communication counseling frequently is an integral part of any clinical interaction. All of these skills can be improved with practice, and they can be applied not only in clinical situations but also in interactions with family and friends or with a counseling partner. They certainly will not detract from already-in-place "people skills" and in fact should enhance them.

## The "Louder" Skills

Dr. Robert Shum, a clinical psychologist with extensive experience in working with families of children with communication disorders, has commented that SLP-As are masters at explaining and informing, but their other counseling skills are not as well developed.[4] My own clinical observations support his view. SLP-As understand their important role in providing facts to families and adults with communication disorders. In some instances, however, information may be presented too early, or it may not be repeated frequently and thus may not be fully understood or useful to the recipients. Of greater importance, many SLP-As appear to think that the louder skills are synonymous with counseling—but this is not the case. These louder skills are merely another aspect of counseling. Because much of the rest of this book is devoted to the acts of teaching, informing, advising, explaining, and planning, no further

---

[4]Van Riper Lecture, Western Michigan University, 2004.

discussion is needed here, except to note that the quieter counseling skills can easily be practiced simultaneously with the louder ones, not only as ends in themselves.

## Final Comments

The completely quiet skills have been saved for last. It is one thing to know what to say. It is quite another to know when to say nothing at all. Meister Eckhard noted in the fifteenth century that "silence is one of the best ways to view God." Being silent, as well as practicing the judicious benefits of pausing, is critical to effective counseling. Much that is beneficial in counseling occurs during the silences and pauses that signal serious contemplation, careful consideration, and deep reflection. The goal of counseling, after all, is not to fill space with sound, but to fill space with sound interaction.

A number of issues that relate to the personal characteristics of skilled counselors are covered in this chapter, which also reviews personal characteristics and attitudes that may typify successful counselors. The material presented is intended to be suggestive, rather than exhaustive. These issues require ongoing consideration; they recur many times throughout this book.

Box 3.10 presents a deceptively simple exercise that nevertheless provides valuable practice with one of the most important listening tools: silence.

---

### Box 3.10 Exercise: The 30-Second Rule*

Practice the 30-Second Rule for conversation for one week. Anytime someone asks a question, wait 30 seconds before answering. Because the pause is obligatory, the likelihood is that the answer will include reflection, examination of intention, and preview of tone—all things that make for a wiser response.

---

*Adapted from Boorstein, S. (1997). *It's Easier Than You Think: The Buddhist Way to Happiness*. New York: HarperCollins.

## References

Battle, D. (Ed.). (2002). *Communication disorders in multicultural populations* (3rd ed.). Boston: Butterworth-Heinemann.

Boorstein, S. (1997). *It's easier than you think: The Buddhist way to happiness*. New York: HarperCollins.

Buber, M. (1958). *I and thou* (2nd ed.) (R. Smith, Trans.). New York: Charles Scribner.

Cassell, E. J. (2005). Compassion. In C. R. Snyder and S. J. Lopez (Eds.), *Handbook of positive psychology* (pp. 434–445). New York: Oxford University Press.

Coulter, A. (1997). Partnerships with patients: The pros and cons of shared decision-making. *Journal of Health Services Research and Policy, 2,* 112–121.

Cousins, N. (1991). *The anatomy of an illness as perceived by the patient*. New York: Bantam, Doubleday.

Fadiman, A. (1997). *The spirit catches you and you fall down*. New York: Farrar, Straus and Giroux.

Frankl, V. (1989). *Man's search for meaning*. New York: Washington Square Press.

Fromm, E. (1947). *Escape from freedom*. New York: Holt.

Gable, S., Reis, H., Impett, E., & Asher, E. (2004). What do you do when things go right? The intrapersonal and interpersonal benefits of sharing good events. *Journal of Personality and Social Psychology, 87,* 228–245.

Gilbert, D. (2006). *Stumbling toward happiness*. New York: Alfred A. Knopf

Goldberg, S. (1997). *Clinical skills for speech-language pathologists*. San Diego, CA: Singular Publishing Group.

Golper, L. A. (1992). *Sourcebook for medical speech-language pathology*. San Diego, CA: Singular Publishing Group

Johnson, A., & Jacobson, B. (1998). *Medical speech-language pathology: A practitioner's guide*. New York: Thieme.

Jordan, L., & Kaiser, W. (1996). *Aphasia: A social approach*. London: Chapman & Hall.

Kockelmann, E., Elger, C. E., & Helmstaedter, C. (2004). Cognitive profile of topiramate as compared with lamotrigine in epilepsy patients on antiepileptic drug polytherapy: Relationships to blood serum levels and co-medication. *Epilepsy and Behavior, 5,* 716–721.

Kuster, J. (2000). Internet resources for stroke and aphasia. *Topics in Stroke Rehabilitation, 7,* 21–31.

Maguire, G. (2000) Impact of antipsychotics on geriatric patients. *Primary Care Companion Journal Clinical Psychiatry, 2,* 166–172.

Papadatou, D. (1997). Training health professionals in caring for dying children and grieving families. *Death Studies, 21,* 575-600.

Payne, J. (1997). *Adult neurogenic language disorders: Assessment and treatment. A comprehensive ethnobiological approach.* San Diego, CA: Singular Publishing Group.

Rao, P. (2006). Emotional intelligence: The sine qua non for a clinical leadership toolbox. *Journal of Communication Disorders, 39,* 310-319.

Reik, T. (1948). *Listening with the third ear.* New York: Noonday Press.

Rogers, C. (1965). *Client-centered therapy.* Boston: Houghton Mifflin.

Rogers, C. (1992). The necessary and sufficient conditions of therapeutic personality change. *Journal of Counseling and Clinical Psychology, 60,* 827-832.

Rogers, S. J. (2004). Developmental regression in autism spectrum disorders. *Mental Retardation and Developmental Disabilities, 10,* 139-143.

Satir, V. (1967). *Conjoint family therapy* (rev. ed.). Palo Alto, CA: Science and Behavior Books.

Schneider, S. (2001). Realistic optimism. *American Psychologist, March,* 250-259.

Simmons-Mackie, N. (2004). Just kidding! Humour and therapy for aphasia. In J. F. Duchan & S. Byng (Eds.), *Challenging aphasia therapies: Broadening the discourse and extending the boundaries.* New York: Psychology Press.

Taylor, B. (2005). Emotional intelligence: A primer for practitioners in human communication disorders. *Seminars in Speech and Language, 2,* 138-148.

Vogel, D., Carter, J., & Carter, P. (1999). *The effects of drugs on communication disorders* (2nd ed.). San Diego, CA: Singular Publishing Group.

Wallace, G. (1993). Adult neurogenic disorders. In D. E. Battle (Ed.), *Communication disorders in multicultural populations.* Boston: Andover Medical Publishers.

Webster, E. (1977). *Counseling parents of handicapped children: Guidelines for improving communication.* New York: Grune & Stratton.

Webster, E., & Newhoff, M. (1981). Intervention with families of communicatively impaired adults. In D. S. Beasley & G. A. Davis (Eds.), *Aging: Communication processes and disorders.* New York: Grune & Stratton.

Worrall, L., & Egan, J. (2000, July 4-7). *Learning to use the Internet: An approach for communicatively-disordered adults.* Poster presented at the Asia Pacific Conference of Speech Pathology and Audiology, Gold Coast, Australia.

# Chapter 4

# COMMUNICATION COUNSELING WITH PARENTS OF CHILDREN AT RISK FOR DISABILITY[1]

*People can live well with any disability if their nations are just, their communities are decent, and their families are supportive and loving. It is OK to be disabled. Disability is not opposed to happiness and quality of life. Why is it that so many of us parents must wait for our children to teach us this fact?*

> Sue Swenson, mother of a child with a severe developmental disability and Executive Director, The Arc of the United States

## Some Fundamentals and Commonalities

It probably is impossible to imagine the overwhelming sense of difficulty and loss for parents who have just begun the process of acknowledging that their newest (perhaps their first) child is not

---

[1] I am grateful to Noel Matkin, PhD, and to Trudi Murch, PhD, for their extensive input into the development of this chapter.

perfect. Few if any children are perfect; nonetheless, all parents have harbored such a secret wish. Parents of children born with disabilities or who are at risk for them face tremendous problems, and their dreams of a perfect child are threatened, if not shattered. This state involves crisis and catastrophe, and the stages of crisis loom large. The first stage is shock that this has happened. Even when the mother has undergone amniocentesis, or when the parents are otherwise forewarned that all might not be well, shock is common to all affected parents. Then comes realization, then perhaps denial, and finally, acknowledgment. Rather than orderly progression from one stage to the next, a more common experience is a mixture of the different stages—perhaps a vacillation between magical thinking directed at the notion that the child has been misdiagnosed (overt denial), or that exceptions occur, or that cures are just around the corner, or that despite the evidence, all will be well (covert denial). These reactions may occur simultaneously with the negativity inherent in having a "damaged child" and what that may mean, not only for the child but also for parents and siblings, for grandparents, and even for society.

This chapter addresses the range of communication problems that burden babies, toddlers, and children up to the age of three or so and their parents. By design, the focus here is on parents. This age range roughly covers the time period during which most counseling efforts should focus on helping parents to get their little ones off to the best possible start. In this time frame, parents are on center stage. Their efforts lay the groundwork that will help their children to live full and satisfying lives. It also is the period of most active language development, when parental input is crucial, and when helping parents to "get it right" at times requires active clinician involvement.

## The Focus Disorders

### Overview

This chapter discusses a number of disorders and at times jumps from one to another for pertinent examples. It focuses on the following categories: severe hearing loss and deafness; cognitive and intellectual disorders, with an emphasis on Down syndrome; autism spectrum disorders; craniofacial anomalies; and cerebral palsy and other neurological disorders that become apparent early in development. Of course, in some cases these disorders overlap. For example, consider the increased likelihood of hearing impairment in conjunction with craniofacial anomalies or Down syndrome. Many other disorders, for example Fragile-X syndrome also can result in communication disabilities, but the examples provided are applicable to them as well.

This is a vast territory. Although the specifics of these disorders differ, they share similar counseling issues, concerns, approaches, and goals. This chapter does not describe the disorders themselves but is concerned with counseling applied to children with such disorders. Your job is to adapt the counseling framework to meet your needs as a clinician and those of the concerned family. A logical place to begin is to consider some differences and similarities among these focus disorders.

## Differences

SLP-As can familiarize themselves with the explicit features of these disorders and the unique direct clinical interventions for them by enrolling in training workshops and the like that are variants on such topics as "Intervention for At-Risk Infants and Children," "Cleft Palate and Craniofacial Anomalies," "Pediatric Audiology," and so on. Generalist SLPs or audiologists who find themselves working in a clinic that specializes in a specific syndrome are expected to avail themselves of all of the books and Internet resources that can enhance their expertise about the disorder.

## Commonalities

The five categories of disorders also have some commonalities, which represent the basic counseling issues. With the possible exception of the high-functioning end of the autism spectrum (e.g., Asperger syndrome), these commonalities are as follows: (1) They all have an early onset, which often comes without warning. (2) All also have enduring effects and typically are chronic. These longstanding effects involve both the children who have the disorders and their families. Satir 1983) referred to the person who carries a particular diagnosis as "the identified patient" in a family, emphasizing in that way the notion that all family members are affected and, to that extent, "patients" as well, only not identified as such. (3) The disorders occur across the economic landscape, but possibly with the exception of autism, they appear to occur disproportionately among less privileged members of society. (4) Finally, all illustrate the importance of early identification and early intervention.

## What Are the Implications for Communication Counseling?

Each of the four commonalities just listed is briefly discussed next.

### *The Shock Factor*

The shock factor has been touched on earlier but certainly bears revisiting. Even parents who have been "prepared" by prenatal counseling may not escape the initial shock of seeing their own child with a craniofacial anomaly, or of knowing that motor development is likely to be different from the norm for their baby with cerebral palsy. Parents frequently are not ready to absorb such information and to move forward. This is catastrophe time, and counselors must be sensitive to the importance and power of grieving, and alert to the likelihood that in many instances, it will take substantial time for parents to be able to process information, suggestions, and so forth. Some problems require direct clinical attention in the earliest phases (for example, adaptations that are necessary for providing adequate nutrition). All require the delicate balance and sensitivity that permits counselors to be good and patient listeners as parents grieve, as well as assisting them in acquiring the information and the accompanying confidence that permits them to start the process of becoming an expert with their own child.

### *The Chronic Factor*

For the disorders that come to clinical attention of SLP-As, counseling involvement increases over the first few years of life. For some problems, other specialists assume the initial burden of helping parents to manage the issue of the chronic conditions that will affect their child and, by extension, their family. Usually by the time SLP-As become intensely involved, chronicity is recognized, if not accepted. Nevertheless, we must be constantly alert to the reality of the lifespan problems many children face, and to the new hurdles that they will face as they mature. It is never prudent to predict outcomes, and communication counselors can never have enough practice with at least 100 variants of "I can't predict." In this regard, it is wise to remember that even a clear statement of uncertainty is much more satisfying than no answer at all. Nevertheless, we must not avoid the issue of chronicity, but use the counseling process to help families face each new hurdle with realistic optimism and resilience. Chapter 8 provides more specific approaches to resilience training.

## *Facing Poverty*

Overwhelmingly, SLP-As in this early part of the twenty-first century come from white, monolingual, middle-class backgrounds. The link between precipitating conditions and poverty basically underscores the fact that most clinicians, regardless of ethnic and cultural backgrounds, will see many families and children who do not necessarily share their predominantly middle class values and upbringing. This difference in backgrounds has at least as many important ramifications for counseling as for direct intervention. Poverty issues require distinct sensitivity to differing realities of living that are likely to have a direct impact on counseling and on interacting with families.

Economic and social class variables are not as well highlighted in our profession's diversity training as are ethnic and cultural variables, or even gender differences. One result of this lack is that economic issues are more insidious than other cross-cultural boundaries for which our training is more explicit. Is Mrs. H late for a session because of a different time perception within her culture, or because of the rigidity of a work schedule that is unsympathetic to the special problems of getting help for an at-risk child? Do one or both parents work two jobs to make ends meet? If so, does child-rearing become a mutual responsibility for a grandparent as a result? Are there special issues with secondary caregivers? Are our referrals within the realm of financial possibility for a given family? If not, how can we as counselors help families to get needed financial help?

### The Need for Early Intervention

Each of the preceding three issues complicates the need for early intervention. For example, if families need time to absorb the catastrophe or if they are denying it, then early intervention may be delayed. If families fail to understand the implications of lifespan problems, they may fail to see the importance of early intervention. It is even possible that the opportunity for early counseling may be missed altogether. After the shock and denial stages comes a daunting task for counselors: to get families to recognize the need for management; to get them to commit to playing a major role in management; and then to guide them in developing a satisfactory implementation plan.

## The Importance of Stories in Counseling Families

The importance of listening to stories probably is never greater in communication counseling than when the stories concern children. As noted earlier, SLPs are seldom the individuals who break the news to families, although audiologists may not get off so easily. In some ways, this suggests that the limited contact that audiologists may have with deaf or hard of hearing children places an extraordinary demand on their counseling skills. Nevertheless, the crucial point is that getting the facts (as in interviewing) or giving the facts (as in providing information) is never enough. Effective counselors who listen to their clients' stories have access to a different, additional database. They listen with an ear to interweaving the stories they hear with planning next steps and ensuring that parents and clinicians understand one another. They also use the stories to help them to get comfortably on the other side of the counseling table and as a result build their own compassion and empathy. Listening to stories, and understanding what they mean to the storyteller, is the major way to begin the process of sharing expertise. Parr, Byng, Gilpin, and Ireland (1997) call such stories "the insider view." Stories are a primary data source. For fully effective counseling, they are as important as the overtly objective data culled from tests and procedures.

And how does one get stories from patients? Although the process lacks the romanticism of journalism, it lacks none of the pleasures. A 2005 interview on National Public Radio (NPR) with Seymour Hersh is revealing. Hersh is the renowned journalist who 40-odd years ago revealed the My Lai Massacre in Vietnam and, more recently (along with CBS), unveiled the tortures at Abu-Ghraib prison (2004). The interviewer asked Mr. Hersh how difficult it was to get credible sources to open up to him, particularly given his reputation as a muckraker. He laughed and replied, "Americans love to talk about what they know, and they are amazingly eager and responsive to being asked."

Comments such as this should encourage communication counselors to "just ask." I often do ask, but I also tend to use directives such as "Tell me your story" or "What's been going on?" or "It would really help me if I knew your story—what you felt and what you were thinking, and that kind of stuff." Box 4.1 contains some additional helpful hints for getting stories.

## What Stories Do

Having an at-risk baby or later realizing that one's toddler turns out to be at risk is a "disorienting dilemma." Thinkers such as Mezirow (1991) have posited that "disorienting dilemmas" may not be totally negative. Rather, they can provide the experienced with an opportunity to rethink, to reconsider, and to rebuild. Mezirow further suggests that disorienting dilemmas can prepare adults for what he calls transformative experiences, resulting in potentially dramatic growth. Having an at-risk child also is the most genuinely catastrophic part of the "whole catastrophe." Telling their story is one way for parents to become more accepting of, perhaps even comfortable with, what has happened to them. Stories repeated often and over time become ways to grow toward acknowledgment.

---

**Box 4.1  The SLP-A as Correspondent: Helpful Hints for Getting the Stories**

- "Help me to understand . . . "
- "What's been happening?"
- "If I'm gonna help you, I need to know what's going on."
- "What's the story?"

---

When stories are shared with others, particularly others whose basic stories are similar, they can become mechanisms for personal growth. Stories can be especially potent when levels of perceived catastrophe are made explicit. When a particularly fragile parent hears a more resilient one describe her own successful coping, the fragile parent may find a role model for growth and resilience.

Parent groups provide a fertile ground for such growth among their members. Communication counselors who hear family stories, who remember the stories of others, and who know the power of such disclosure also can be effective in helping parents who are unable to participate in groups. In such cases, the clinician serves as the "surrogate mouthpiece" for many other people, including those whose experiences that are documented in books and testimonials. A clinician with a sharp memory and a well-honed bibliography is a rich resource for families. This underscores the necessity of keeping up to date in the search for good stories, books, or films to share.

## Understanding Parents' Perspectives

Most clinicians probably make some implicit assumptions concerning what it means to be a "good parent." These assumptions may be based on our own mothers or fathers, or those of friends, or perhaps a composite of TV-character moms, with a bit of Catherine Zeta-Jones and Miss Holbrook, our cherished second-grade teacher, built in. This composite is the "good parent" whom we would aspire to be. Not surprisingly, most parents we work with also have implicit assumptions and aspirations concerning themselves as parents. How those aspirations are framed may differ, but they help us to understand the various faces of parenting.

My own "good parent" role model was focused primarily on helping my kids to become autonomous—to develop their own goals for their lives, to define their societal responsibilities, to develop their own models for "success." Other parents may see their role as helping their children to fit in, or to become financially successful, or to develop values in tune with the family's religious traditions, and so forth. No one view is right or wrong—views are just different.

There are also less carefully delineated views. For example, the model may be something like "I want to be just like my mother" or, conversely, "I want to be just the opposite of my parents." Finding out what good parenting means to a mother or father is basic to providing appropriate counseling. It's important for the clinician-counselor to refrain from trying to change values; rather, all values should be respected. One aspect of parent counseling is to help parents to understand their own aspirations, to follow their own dreams, and to make appropriate modifications when their child differs from their expectations. The "child who might have been" is possibly a ghost in the treatment room.

This idea of a ghost, present but not visible, comes from an influential parenting essay by Fraiberg, Adlson, and Shapiro: "Ghosts in the Nursery" (1975). The ghosts in this essay are one's own parents and their often unrecognized and unseen influences on an individual's parenting styles. But there may be others, such as the "child who might have been" just mentioned. How does the communication counselor find out which ghosts are affecting parents? First, of course, is by listening intently with all three ears, and next, by questioning, re-stating, confirming, and so forth when necessary.

A final comment before moving on: Communication counselors rely on their own understanding of the normal language acquisition process to guide and to help parents understand what is going on with their children. This is an important counseling responsibility, but it should be supplemented with readable, lay-oriented material about normal language as well. Box 4.2 lists some books that meet this need.

---

### Box 4.2 Books on Language Acquisition

Acredolo, L., & Goodwin, S. (2002). *Baby signs: How to talk with your baby before your baby can talk to you.* Lincolnwood, IL: NTC Publishing.

Apel, K., & Masterson, J. J. (2001). *Beyond baby talk: From sounds to sentences: A parent's complete guide to language development.* Roseville, CA: Prima Publishing.

Golinkoff, R. M., & Hirsh-Pasek, K. (1999). *How babies talk: The magic and mystery of language in the first three years.* New York: Dutton/Penguin Press.

Hirsh-Pasek, K., & Golinkoff, R. M., with Eyer, D. (2003). *Einstein never used flash cards: How our children really learn and why they need to play more and memorize less.* Emmaus, PA: Rodale Press.

## What Big Issues Do Parents Worry About?

Doris and Harry, the parents of a child with Down syndrome, reported that when they became aware of their baby daughter Sarah's condition, they immediately developed fears for their marriage and the effects Sarah would have on it. For example, was the marriage strong enough to withstand the unplanned-for stresses and strains that they both believed were inevitable consequences of Sarah's disability? Were there new financial burdens on their horizon? Next, they expressed fears for their other children, Dan and Gwen. How would Sarah affect her siblings' lives? Would Doris and Harry have enough time to parent them all three of them effectively? The money question was again raised, as were simple fears about how accepting Gwen and Dan would be of their baby sister.

Such worries and fears were the background against which fears for Sarah herself began to emerge. Doris and Harry summarized their fears for Sarah as follows: They worried about Sarah's acceptance by others and her happiness. They worried about her safety. They feared that she would never be independent. Box 4.3 restates them.

Although the goals of acceptance, safety, independence, and happiness have been cast here in the framework of Down syndrome, they can as easily be applied to the wide range of disorders that occur very early in life.

A third look should reveal that Doris and Harry have cast a very wide net indeed. Are these not the aspirations of all parents for their children? There may be nuances and differences relative to one's culture and circumstances, but such goals, and worries concerning their achievement, are universal, not just about children at risk for handicap.

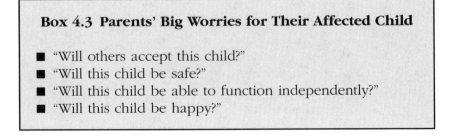

**Box 4.3 Parents' Big Worries for Their Affected Child**

- "Will others accept this child?"
- "Will this child be safe?"
- "Will this child be able to function independently?"
- "Will this child be happy?"

## What Do Parents Worry About? The Smaller Issues and Counseling Moments

Although framed by the large issues, the details of the smaller issues are devilish as well. For example, Alison and Rich, whose son Scott has moderately severe cerebral palsy, have many small worries. Although they share the classic larger worries for parents of children with disabilities, Alison and Rich are focusing on smaller ones, such as those that appear in Box 4.4. Questions such as these are often asked point blank to clinicians who work with children. In my experience, such smaller worries are the ones that provide communication counselors with some of the *counseling moments* introduced in Chapter 1 in the form of questions that may occur before a clinical session with a child gets under way, or at its termination. Box 4.4 provides a sampling.

Far more frequently than specific sessions set aside to talk it over, or to furnish information, counseling moments provide communication counselors with excellent opportunities to be of help to parents. To take advantage of them, the counselor must first be on the lookout for their appearance, and then be responsive to them. Sometimes a question concerning a relatively less important question may signal the presence of a much bigger issue, whereas at other times such questions may indicate the need for simple reassurance. For example, the time management issue is universal

---

### Box 4.4 Parents' Immediate Worries for Managing Life with Their Affected Child

- "Do you think I am a good parent to this child?"
- "How do I manage my time?"
- "How do I discipline this toddler?"
- "How do I explain him to others?"
- "How do I avoid playing favorites with my kids?"
- "Where do I get everyday advice?"
- "What about our other kids?"
- "What about me?"

and for some parents can be addressed with joint problem-solving work. For others, the time management question may be a way to discover whether they are adequate parents. (This is just a reminder to stay alert for latent content.) Box 4.5 contains some examples of questions from parents about issues that may or may not fall within the SLP-A's scope of practice

A useful way to practice management of counseling moments is to keep a small notebook with you during your days in the clinic. As such moments occur, not only to you but to your colleagues, jot them down, along with their consequences. Then spend time later evaluating how effective the interchanges were, and how they might have been improved.

Another fruitful exercise is to develop lists of interesting clinical dilemmas and to come up with after-the-fact ideas of how they might have been differently, perhaps even better, handled. This type of "Monday morning quarterbacking" often can be helpful when similar situations arise in the future. Box 4.6 provides a sampling for practice.

## A Final Thought on Parent Perspectives

It is important to emphasize that "special needs" children are perhaps not so special after all. They are part of the fabric of life (the "full catastrophe"), and the normal parental aspirations for happiness of the child apply. They are, first and most basically, children, not disabled children. This idea is perhaps the most fundamental on which to build a realistic and healthy foundation for a positive life—for the child, for the parents, and for the family as a whole.

## Some Specific Words about Specifics

Specific facts about the disorders we work with have powerful influences on communication counseling. It is inappropriate here to review the full breadth of knowledge that affects the counseling process, because such knowledge, both of the disorders and of their specific interventions, has been basic to formal coursework in the study of human communication and its disorders.

## Box 4.5 Exercise: Scope of Practice Boundaries with Specific Clinical Scenarios

The following comments from parents of at-risk infants and toddlers each define a specific clinical scenario. As the clinician in each case, decide whether the resulting "counseling moment" is within your scope of practice. If it is not, then answer from that perspective. If you decide it is within your scope of practice, answer from that perspective. Try for more than one answer. Feel free to add relevant context.

"How can you discipline a 2-year-old who doesn't understand you?"

"She takes up so much of my time and energy that I'm close to ignoring my other kids."

"We really can't decide on the pros and cons of a cochlear implant for Louie. What should we do?"

"I wish I could figure it out. Nothing like this ever happened to me before. I don't think I can manage this baby!

"We just found out the most amazing thing! They've found that there is a link between eating bananas and autism. We have already stopped eating them, and I think I can see a difference in Frances already! What do you think?"

"I really am a nervous wreck. I lie awake and worry if he's even getting enough to eat, and every time he cries, I just go all to pieces."

"Can you help us think of something to do that might help my wife and me to feel a little better about ourselves?"

"If I have to remind Tom once more to pay some attention to his little brother, I think I'll scream. Tom would be better with him if Teddy didn't have CP, I feel sure."

"Am I really an okay mom? How do other parents do it?"

"My wife Suzy thinks this problem is with the genes on my side of the family, and I'm to blame. I wish I knew how to deal with that."

**Box 4.6**
**Exercise: Clinical Dilemmas**

1. Ashton is an autistic 5-year-old. Today, when you were seeing him for language therapy, he bit you on the arm, not hard enough to break the skin through your long-sleeved sweater, but enough leave a bruise. Ashton's mother was observing the session through a one-way mirror and saw the incident.

   ■ What do you do with Ashton?
   ■ What do you say to his mother?

   In another version of this scenario, Ashton's mother was not observing at the time and thus missed the incident. You knew she was not there.

   ■ Does this change what you do with Ashton, or his mother?
   ■ If yes, state the alternatives.

2. Camille is a 4-year-old child with moderate cerebral palsy. Her mother accompanies her to the therapy room, and when she leaves, Camille begins to cry. You attempt to distract her, but after 10 minutes, you make no discernible progress.

   ■ What do you do next?
   ■ What do you say to Camille's mother?

   At another session, you manage successfully to distract Camille, and she stops crying after a few minutes. At the end of the session, Camille's mother says to you: "How did you do that? It never seems to work for me at home!"

   ■ What do you do or say?

Some facts and some questions, however, are at the heart of the communication counseling process and are quite specific to the roles of informing, advising, and teaching. Some of the most important are discussed next, along with a strategy for obtaining the minimum information that a dedicated counselor should have at his or her fingertips.

## What Information Do Communication Counselors Need about the Disorders They Will Encounter in Clinical Practice?

The first responsibility of clinician-counselors who take jobs in a center that focuses on treatment of a condition about which they have little information is to augment their knowledge with as with as much relevant information as possible. This information should come from a number of sources: books, colleagues, videotapes, websites, parents, and community resources. It is important to be up to date on professional resources, as well as to know the more general literature or websites that parents may have already visited, or that can be recommended to them. This information, of course, will apply fundamentally to the evaluation and treatment of a specific disorder. But a substantial amount of it applies to the counseling aspects of the disorders as well.

Following is a list of essential questions for which parents will need answers:.

- What are the genetic characteristics of Disorder A?

  If the parents have other children, are they likely to have this disorder?

  If they have other children who do *not* have this disorder, why not?

  What are the risks for their children as future parents concerning Disorder A?

- If not genetics, then what?

  Did I [the mother] fail to take care of some aspect of my health? Did I do something wrong?

  Are we being punished for past misdeeds?

  Did it just happen? How satisfying is such an explanation?

- What is the developmental course of Disorder A?

  What future problems can be foreseen?

  What potential problems can be forestalled?

  What does the future hold?

- Do other problems accompany the communication disorder?

  If so, what are they?

- Where is help to be found?
- What about support groups?
- What other options are there for treatment? How can I know which will help?

This is only a sampling of relevant questions. They are not meant to encourage communication counselors to overstep the American Speech-Language-Hearing Association (ASHA) Scope of Practice and pretend to be medical experts or genetic counselors, or early childhood education specialists. Rather, they underscore the need for communication counselors to have up-to-date genetic information or, for non-genetically related disorders, explicitly current medical and pharmacological information in case they are called on to clarify or to repeat what the real experts have said. They also illustrate the tremendous advantage that accrues when SLP-As collaborate with specialists from other disciplines.

It also is important to listen for when parents have misunderstood. In such instances, we can help by referring parents back to the appropriate information sources for clarification and further explanation. To be an effective broker of such information, astute counselors need as much information about parental beliefs as possible, as well as the facts. It is important to recognize that such beliefs often are culturally influenced and may vary widely.

## How Might This All Play Out? A Strategy

Because my career has centered largely on work with adults, I have not acquired the in-depth knowledge of basic child disorders that characterizes SLP-As who work predominantly with children. I decided it would be instructive for me to try to catch up on some of the disorders to which I had paid little attention over the years and for which the explosions in medical and genetic knowledge had left my knowledge base far behind. My plan was to use my adventures to illustrate a workable strategy for how to play catch-up.

The result was about eight pages of truly "show-off" text about the genetics of Usher's and Waardenburg's syndromes and lots more about mirror neurons, theory of mind, and so on. The specifics of what I learned probably will never come to clinical application with my clients, who typically have post-stroke aphasia. It is the *strategy* I used to acquire my updated knowledge that's of relevance here.[2] I tried to conduct my research in a manner similar to what families might use: I sought out experts; I went to the popular, self-help press; and I spent hours on the Internet. All were rewarding.

The Internet offers a surprising amount of solid, corroborated information about all of the focus disorders in this chapter. Nonetheless, not all of the information I found was useful or even correct. For example, one site stated that Waardenburg's syndrome resulted from a recessive gene (not true, it appears to be a dominant trait). I champion the Internet and use it frequently. Nevertheless, it is mandatory for communication counselors to validate sources, and also to warn parents about possible inconsistencies on the Internet, as well as its sometimes unfounded pronouncements and misinformation. A few of the most useful, but far from exhaustive, Internet sources are listed at the end of the chapter.

I also learned about some issues concerning etiologies and treatments for various disorders that had emerged and some that had dissipated over the past years. I knew, as will most readers, that Kanner's "Iceberg Mom" (1979) had melted, and could no longer be held responsible for creating autistic children of course,[3] because of earlier reading related to my obsession with the brain. But in the meantime, other sources of potential parental guilt appear to have intensified. Three examples related to congenital disabilities are illustrative: fetal alcohol syndrome (FAS), infants born to mothers who have been taking isoretinoin (Accutane) to treat severe acne, and the congenital problems of babies who are born with human immunodeficiency virus (HIV) infection. Counseling issues that result for such parents may include dealing not only with immediate parental guilt but also with persisting aftereffects.

---

[2]The information I compiled generally was accurate, as reviewed by pediatric neurologist Katherine Holland, MD (my daughter).

[3]The cautionary tale is that communication counselors must stay up to date. Because we have the power to help, we also have the power to harm, and we must be mindful of this. One way to harm is to let our information gather dust and rust. Think of the damage I could have done if I never updated what was a perfectly acceptable answer to a comprehensive examination question when I was in school.

## Some Things That Haven't Changed Very Much: The Course of the Disorder

Usher syndrome, along with some other disorders, has a particularly grim prognosis. Accordingly, communication counselors may need to think through the implications for counseling in cases involving such disorders, and to decide how much information to provide and when to provide it. No rules exist, but it is a good practice is to provide as much information the family can handle. Some parents may want a lifespan perspective (a difficult challenge, of course); others want to find out only what they need to know for tomorrow. Parental needs should be honored to the extent possible.

Regardless of the extent of the information the communications counselor provides, it is never a "one-stop service." Matkin suggests that audiologists who inform parents about hearing problems in their children should initially schedule at least two sessions (N. D.Matkin, personal communication, 2006). The first session is to break the news. The second session, preferably undertaken a week or so later, has two goals: (1) to establish what information the parents have correctly or incorrectly absorbed, and to clear up misunderstandings, and (2) to begin developing an active habilitation plan. These goals constitute just the beginning. A rigorous schedule of counseling probably is needed during early preschool years— about every 6 months for the first 3 years and then every year until age 6. Particularly for hearing disorders and perhaps specific language impairment (SLI), for which counselors are likely to be the first bearers of definitive bad news, crisis theory suggests that acknowledgment of the problem often takes time. Information about course and outcome probably has to be revisited frequently, regardless of who breaks the bad news. What's down the road engenders anxiety and possibly depression, and the extent to which communication counselors are able to allay them is of great value.

Finally, it must be noted that sometimes the etiological explanations and treatments that are attractive to families fall far short of providing convincing evidence to clinicians and scientists. Websites and books that fervently promulgate unproven causes and treatments may influence parents. This is a counseling issue, and it threatens the concept of mutual expertise that is a key precept of the clinical approach developed in this book.

Helping parents to stay focused on the problem and its solutions and not on its cause could well be a slogan for all of us to embrace. We need to handle all of these issues while remaining current and open-minded concerning rapidly growing and potentially changing etiological evidence.

## What Are the Accompanying Problems?

When I asked a graduate class in counseling to describe their most nightmarish client, I expected them to discuss individuals with communication disorders, such as an adult with primary progressive aphasia, or perhaps an adolescent who stutters. Instead, the students, to a person, described their nightmare clients not by their communication disorders or their age, but by their "alongside problems."

*Alongside problems* are not the expected cognitive or behavioral concomitants of many of the disorders, such as retardation, pragmatic problems, or attention deficit disorder, or even sensory and motor accompaniments. My students rightly noted that they had been well prepared through their coursework for those things. Instead, they described problems that fell into two general categories: (1) unwieldy emotional responses in young clients and (2) interpersonal issues with their young clients' parents. Such problems tend to tax our counseling skills, perhaps because they present situations in which clinicians may feel that they are ineffective and inadequate as a result of their lack of training in managing them. Solutions relate to counseling skills.

Many alongside problems also embody parent anxiety, confusion, and bewilderment about parenting children with disabilities. They may concern issues in behavior management, realized in possibly unspoken questions such as "How can I guide Sean in appropriate behavior when he can't understand me?" or "Who could possibly discipline Nina, with all her physical disabilities?" (See Box 4.4.)

Related alongside issues also may include the extent of trust that parents feel they can confidently place in clinicians who have a large number of children on their caseloads. That is, do Maria's parents trust her clinician to be sensitive to their daughter's special needs? After all, Maria is at the very center of her parents' maelstrom and perhaps represents only a ripple in the water for her clinician. Another parent may wonder, "How can I be sure that any clinician will understand Josh's needs if I am not there to interpret? After all, he has a communication problem."

The sadness and sense of loss that frequently accompany the unexpected presence of a handicapped child not only produce bewilderment but also can result in parental depression. With depression, the ability to parent effectively is likely to be compromised. This impairment may affect both children with disabilities and their non-handicapped siblings. Maintaining alertness to depression and anxiety is a constant responsibility of SLP-As.

Finally, there is frequently a cross-cultural component to parental trust. If cross-cultural issues appear to be adversely influencing the counseling relationship, it is imperative that the counselor take the initiative for resolving them, whether by referral, by attempts at open discussion, or by seeking additional help.

SLP-As are not expected to be parenting specialists. Nevertheless, they must be exquisitely sensitive to such general issues if they are to be effective clinicians. SLPs must be strong enough to point out children's inappropriate behaviors to parents, particularly if those behaviors have a negative effect on clinical interaction and outcome. Furthermore, if clinicians see parental behavior as the root of their child's problem behavior, they must deal with this as well. To develop the ability to address these issues, clinicians can incorporate several practices into their interactions with parents:

- Practicing diplomacy, preferably by learning to be diplomatic in relation to less thorny problems
- Listening patiently and well, and using the listening process to pinpoint the root of the problem
- Managing any personal sense of hurt, or anger, or injustice
- Being knowledgeable about parenting resources, as well as ready and willing to refer
- Taking risks and rising to challenges

This aspect of communication counseling is a challenging but fulfilling one.

## Helping Parents to Find Help and to Advocate

Jacob is a child with autism. His father has written extensively about Jacob's management for the website www.zerotothree.org. To professionals who might work with Jacob and his family, Jacob's dad gave the following advice:

> Help parents, be sensitive to our needs, but remember who the client is. Don't let us off the hook. Push us, challenge us, keep us on task. We must be a main protagonist if our child is going to get better.
>
> In many communities, the structures and services have not caught up with current innovations and new approaches to intervention. Empower us to be advocates on behalf of our children and embolden us to be subversive when we need to be.
>
> Knowledge and understanding will empower us. Confusion and lack of clarity are disabling. Take the time to explain the issues to us with words we will understand.
>
> Finally, incremental changes in practice and perceptions will not suffice. Rather, a radical paradigm shift concerning the fundamental assumptions regarding who these children with severe disorders in relating and communicating are and what they can accomplish is called for. (From: "Jacob's Story: A Miracle of the Heart," by "Jacob's Father," edited from a special edition of the April/May 1997 Zero to Three Journal. www.zerotothree.org. Reprinted with permission.)

As eloquently stated by Jacob's father, a basic responsibility of communication counselors is to help parents in their quest for the help they perceive they need, and to help them become advocates for their children. As discussed previously, communication counselors are obligated to know the resources available in the community. Particularly important, of course, are parent groups and the opportunities they present for encouraging parents to learn not only from professionals but also from each other.

## The Internet

As noted, the Internet is increasingly important for parents as they seek information pertinent to managing their children's disabilities. Especially useful and reliable sources of such information are the various websites provided by the National Institute of Mental Health (NIMH) and National Institutes of Health (NIH), particularly the websites of the National Institute of Child Health and Development (NICHD) and the National Institute of Deafness and Other

Communication Disorders (NIDCD), and those of advocacy organizations such as United Cerebral Palsy, The Arc of the United States, and Family Village, an international resource for persons with disabilities.

## Networks and Support Groups

Equally important are the growing networks of parent support groups, and the information that parents provide for each other through these networks. A look at self-help websites makes it abundantly clear that many parents have earned their designations as experts in the disorders that affect their children. A sampling of parent support and advocacy websites is provided at the end of the chapter. The listing is not exhaustive in terms of either the problems covered or the extent of good coverage for frequently occurring conditions. An important consideration is that websites must be constantly checked for updates, changes, accuracies, even disappearances. The listing for this chapter merely includes those that currently are among the most parent friendly and provide honest, and uplifting and positive information. These websites are easy for parents to access and to participate in their chat rooms and blogsites.

## A Model of Advocacy

Sue Swenson is the Director of the Arc of the United States, devoted to advocacy and support for persons who have cognitive and intellectual disorders and for their families. The following account of her own experience as the mother of a child with a disability (reproduced from an Arc newsletter, in slightly abridged form) gives her vision of advocacy, which should prove instructive for any counselor who works with parents of children with disabilities.

> When my son Charlie was a baby, the doctor said he was "developmentally delayed." This was a comfort to me, oddly, after months of asking, "What is wrong?" and being told, "There is nothing wrong. Don't compare him to his brother." I didn't know what "developmental delay" meant, but it seemed to mean that I was right to ask if something was wrong. That was a comfort.

The doctor sent me to a brilliant therapist, who told me the truth—that my son's delays were very "significant," that no one could know how everything would turn out, that there were many ways to help him play and have fun with other kids so that his development would not be so affected by his obvious problems. I thought that by talking about hope for his development, she was telling me Charlie's "delays" might go away. I could not imagine and did not have the experience to image that there could be hope *with* disabilities.

When Charlie was seven, . . . it hit me like a thunderbolt: Charlie's "delays" were not going to go away, and instead of therapy aimed at "fixing" him, he needed inclusive education to make sure that he could make the most out of learning opportunities. He would not be "ready" for school as his classmates are ready. But he needed to stop trying to learn stuff that was difficult or impossible to master, like tying his shoes, so that he could move on and learn the important stuff, like how to get along with other people. You can buy shoes with Velcro closures, but there is no Velcro to help you form human attachments.

. . . It is so hard to find the right words to use when talking to parents about disability in children. The future holds so much potential, so much uncertainty, and so much fear. Usually, we parents don't know what it is like to be disabled in America. Unlike most other minorities, we don't often share our child's identifying characteristics.

In my experience, glossing disability over and calling it "delay" doesn't help. It makes parents think that in the end, if we work hard enough, everything will be OK because in the end our child will "catch up." When we are focused on catching up, we don't work on justice for people with disabilities because we don't let ourselves think our children will actually be disabled when they grow up.

No matter what we are told, I think most of us know in our hearts that disabilities are real, and persistent. We, and our children, can be hurt by not letting ourselves think about that reality. We need to learn that hoping, praying, suing, or paying for a "cure" takes away precious time from the real goals of teaching our children that we love them as they are, of helping our children learn how to live well with their disability, and of helping our communities rise to the challenge of justice, decent support and equal access.

Too many children keep getting therapy to help them walk while they get no instruction in how to use a wheelchair;

too many keep trying to develop the muscles they need to speak while they get no evaluation for a communication device; too many children spend their school day going from therapy to therapy instead of making friends in their classroom. Too often, children live like this because their parents can't or won't or haven't been encouraged to accept the reality of disability.

Parent advocates have two paths before us: (1) We can use all of our power and parental rights to deny the impending reality of disability, to demand enough therapy to make the "delays" go away; or (2) we can use our voice and our rights to demand justice, access and inclusion for all of our sons and daughters, and to demand recognition of their rights as human beings and as citizens *with* disabilities. For most parents, advocacy will be a mix of these. Mine was—but experience tells me that it is far better to focus on the latter.

In my experience, many young adults with disabilities are still hoping for their parents to make this leap. In my experience, too many feel their parents are somehow disappointed by their disability, and they feel a righteous anger about this.

We can help our kids if we understand that our sons and daughters are people with disabilities not "delays," and that people with disabilities are people first—*whole* people first. The sooner have a chance to learn this, the sooner we can clear up any confusion in our relationships with our children, and the sooner we can say to them, honestly and truthfully: "I see you as you are. I love you as you are. I am proud of you as you are. I will do whatever I can to help you be the best you possible, and I will insist on recognition of your rights."

Maybe then our children can love us as we are, too, although we don't know everything they need to learn, and can't fix everything that may trouble them in life." (*Newsletter of The Arc of the United States*, 2004. Reprinted with permission.)

## Moving On

Until Jacob and Charlie's parents talked about their experiences, this chapter emphasized unpleasant, sad, and depressing issues. This has not been totally encouraging from a positive psychology perspective. Chapter 8 focuses on a model for communication counselors to follow in helping parents and families build optimism and resilience to counteract the problems described in this and subsequent chapters. Here the contributions of two more parents of children with disabilities, whose work on behalf of their cause has been both highly effective and inspiring, are described. They also serve as paragons for the power of a positive frame of mind.

Louise Tracy is a prime example. An amazing feature of her work is that it occurred long before the advent of the disability movement, and in many ways in isolation from other philanthropists. Her tireless devotion to the education and development of her son John, who was born with a severe hearing impairment, resulted in the development of the prestigious John Tracy Clinic in Los Angeles.

A more recent example is Cynthia Kidder of the Band of Angels Foundation and founder of the Band of Angels Press. She is not a psychologist, nor is she formally educated in positive psychology. She is a doer and builder and responder to challenge, and she is committed to changing the world. She also is an everyday hero whose character strengths include optimism, bravery, and the ability to love and be loved. Along with Brian Skotko, she is the author of *Common Threads: Celebrating Life with Down Syndrome* (2001). The book is positive psychology embodied.

*Common Threads* includes beautiful photographs of children with Down syndrome (photographed by Kendra Dew) accompanied by inspiring stories of their lives as artists, brothers and sisters, learners, athletes, and friends. Children from a variety of backgrounds and situations are included, and the "common thread" in the book's title is inclusion and acceptance. Following is a note from the book's flyleaf, about Kidder, her family, and her life:

> Cynthia is the mother of three boys, one of whom has Down syndrome. Since his birth in 1989, she has devoted her professional energies to providing positive images and opportunities for people with Down syndrome and other differences. As founder of the Band of Angels Press, she has been publishing calendars and cards featuring children and young adults with Down syndrome since 1995. She notes, "I want the world to see not the differences, but the sameness of children and adults with disabilities." (from the flyleaf of *Common Threads* by C. Kidder and B. Skotko2001, Band of Angels Press. Reprinted with permission.)

And from the website:

> When my husband and I were given the news that our new-born son had Down syndrome, I knew my life was changed forever. I worried about everything and thought too much about his future. I thought he belonged to a category of people I didn't understand. Only when I held him did I allow him simply to be my son. That was when his magic took hold. I prized academic achievement; his father prized athletic accomplishments; clearly Jordan would follow in neither my academic nor his father's athletic footsteps. But oh, what a trail he has made! His own footsteps blaze forth in a way that harms no one and charms everyone. He has taught us to be more patient with our older sons when they get imperfect report cards or search for four-leaf clovers while playing left field.
>
> Certainly life has been different, but the irony is this: Life has been better since Jordan than we ever could have imagined. We enjoy more of life's details. We listen to the wind. We laugh easily. We know how little we really know about predicting happiness for any of our children. When I look back at those early days and the anxiety we had for our children's future, I wish we had more information that was positive. What we received was so pessimistic and clinical. The pictures in the book I received were of children who had been institutionalized and had no sparkle in their eyes. But in my Jordan's eyes was not some disappointing syndrome but pure sparkle. (www.Bandofangels.com. Reprinted with permission.)

The website (www.bandofangels.com) is luminous. It contains calendars and notepapers featuring children with Down syndrome, inspirational milestone books for parents, a few chat rooms for families and siblings, and fine stories about the Kidder family's growing up with Jordan.

## Conclusions

At a recent conference on adult communication disorders held in St. Louis MO, Joseph Duffy, PhD, of the Mayo Clinic in Rochester, MN described the potential for a crucial role of SLP-As in the differential diagnosis of medical conditions that create disorders such as dysarthria, not just in the differential diagnosis of the dysarthria itself.. He emphasized the importance of going beyond describing what we see, being professionally responsible enough to challenge physicians whose knowledge of speech and language may be insufficient for them to note the consistent patterns that, say, distinguish the dysarthria of a person with myasthenia gravis from the dysarthria of a person who has amyotrophic lateral sclerosis (ALS), with their different treatments and outcomes. In a discussion session following the speech, a number of people in the audience expressed concern that such direct involvement regarding the details of a medical diagnosis was beyond the scope of practice for SLPs. Dr. Duffy affirmed that we do not and should not make medical diagnoses, but emphasized that it is our responsibility to state, when we can, if a particular communication disorder is, could be, or is not compatible with a given medical diagnosis. Thus, if we "disagree" with a physician, we are not disputing the medical diagnosis; rather we are simply noting whether the speech-language problem is or is not compatible with it.

In the context of clinical practice, Dr. Duffy's approach clearly differentiates the carpenter from the craftsperson, the technician from the scientist. Developing a professional identity that supports the latter roles is a key element of a wellness approach to counseling. For communication counselors, the difference between being a capable clinician and a truly gifted one lies in the care with which we augment our clinical skill with our counseling talents. This constitutes a direct application of the "Duffy approach": Our counseling sensitivity turns us from carpenters into craftspeople, and from technicians into clinical scientists. These are roles wherein we will find our deepest personal satisfaction—and, of greater importance, our clients can be expected to reap maximal benefits from our interventions.

# References

Duffy, J. (2006). Differential diagnosis of dysarthria. Paper presented at the Midwest Aphasia and Cognitive Disorders Group (MACDG), September 30, 2006, St. Louis MO.

Fraiberg, S., Adelson, E., & Shapiro, V. (1975). Ghosts in the nursery: A psychoanalytic approach to the problem of impaired infant-mother relationships. *Journal of the American Academy of Child Psychiatry, 14,* 799–803.

"Jacob's Father." (1997). *Jacob's story: A miracle of the heart.* Edited from the April/May Zero to Three Journal, www.zerotothree.org

Kanner, L. (1979). *Child psychiatry.* Smithfield, IL: Charles C Thomas.

Kidder, C. & Skotko, B. (2001). *Common threads: Celebrating life with Down syndrome.* Rochester Hills, MI: Band of Angels Press.

Mezirow, J. (1991). *Transformative dimensions of adult learning.* San Francisco: Jossey-Bass.

Parr, S., Byng, S., Gilpin, S, & Ireland, C. (1997). *Talking about aphasia: Living with loss of language following stroke.* Buckingham, UK: Open University Press.

Satir, V. (1983). *Conjoint family therapy* (3rd ed.). Palo Alto, CA: Science and Behavior Books.

Swenson, S. (2004). Newsletter of the Arc of the United States.

## Websites

The following websites were chosen primarily because they are those of advocacy groups or otherwise addressed to parents, and because they provide links to other websites of interest. Only a few sites per disorder are provided, although there are many more. Using a search engine such as Google and entering the relevant search term for each disorder listed here, as well as many others, will yield specific technical information. Generally, such information is clearly available under the refined search term "health professionals." Communication counselors should be particularly careful to check websites periodically for their relevance, factual content, and currency. Also, it is important to pay frequent visits to the various NIH/NIMH* websites for updates.

### Focus Disorders

Autism spectrum disorders

www.kylestreehouse.org

www.maapservices.org

Cerebral palsy

www.originsofcerebralpalsy.com

www.ucp.org

---

*National Institutes of Health/National Institute of Mental Health.

Cleft palate and other craniofacial anomalies

    www.widesmiles.org

    www.apert.org

    www.faces-cranio.org

    www.friendlyfaces.org

Down syndrome

    www.ndss.org

    www.bandofangels.com

## Hearing

    www.handsandvoices.org

    http://www.beginningssvcs.com

## General

    www.familyvillage.wisconsin.edu

    www.thearc.org

    www.zerotothree.org

# Chapter 5

# COUNSELING ISSUES WITH CHILDREN AND ADOLESCENTS WITH LATER-DEVELOPING COMMUNICATION DISORDERS

## Written in collaboration with Patrick Finn, PhD

"*Dakota*" was a 16-year-old high school student when she wrote the following account of her early life experiences as a young person who stutters:

> After my sixth grade year, I decided that I couldn't let my stuttering stop me any more. I was going to junior high school in a few months and it was time to start being like all the other kids.
>
> Then, two years ago I joined the marching band at my high school. We went to band camp, and I met a lot of new people, and nobody paid attention to my stuttering. This was the first time in my life that people didn't treat me different

because of my stuttering. That was also when I realized that my stuttering really didn't matter to other people. In fact, my band teacher had been my teacher for two years and didn't even know I stuttered until just this past year.

Now that I'm in high school, I really don't enjoy getting up in front of people and giving speeches, but everyone has to do some things in life they don't want to do. I love to talk. I spend most of my time out of school on the phone, and I've made a whole lot of friends. I'm now very outspoken. I don't hide any of my emotions anymore. I tell people what's on my mind, and when I want to talk, I do.

When I'm having a bad day, I stutter more than I do when I have a good day. But sometimes days go by when I don't stutter at all, and it makes me feel great.

I hope this letter inspires many people my age. I hope younger children can learn that they are not the only ones out there who stutter, and that they can stand up for themselves. I had a fantastic speech teacher when I was in elementary school. She was willing to listen to what I had to say, and she taught me how to deal with my stuttering. She was a great person.

Don't worry if people make fun of you. They can't help it. I used to get angry when people would laugh at me, but that's one thing you just have to ignore in life. Don't let anyone tell you that you can't do something because you stutter; you can do whatever you feel like doing and saying. My stuttering used to have a great impact on my life, but now I have learned to work around it. (Reproduced with permission from the National Stuttering Association)

## Introduction

This chapter focuses on children in whom communication problems that were not forecast during their infancy and toddlerhood developed later on, in preschool or kindergarten or even during adolescence—that is, after normal speech and language acquisition was well under way. Many of its concepts also are relevant to children with the focus disorders covered in Chapter 4, and their families, as they grow older. In this chapter, counseling settings are expanded to include schools and clinicians who work there; counseling involves direct work with children in addition to families.

# The Focus Disorders and Their Similarities

Because a complete review of all later-onset communication problems is not possible here, two specific disorders serve as exemplars: stuttering and traumatic brain injury (TBI). TBI and stuttering have commonalities and differences that between them encompass the range of childhood communication counseling issues, from specific language impairment (SLI) to voice and phonological disorders and to rare syndromes.

Box 5.1 summarizes the shared and distinctive attributes of stuttering and TBI that pinpoint the relevant counseling issues. (As an exercise, choose another later-developing disorder such as SLI. Consider what attributes listed for both stuttering and TBI also apply for the third disorder.)

## The Late Factor

All late-developing disorders, including phonological problems and SLI, share a characteristic that distinguishes the affected families and children from those discussed in Chapter 4. Specifically, for all of them, parents have observed some normal language development, and perhaps they breathed a sigh of relief about how well things are going. They've probably formed a rudimentary vision of

---

### Box 5.1 Similarities and Differences: The Counseling Menu for Stuttering and TBI

| Counseling Issue | Stuttering | TBI |
| --- | --- | --- |
| Time of detection | late | late |
| Outcome | unclear | unclear |
| Severity | wide range | wide range |
| Fluctuations | great | small |
| Etiology | unclear | clear |
| Accompanying problems | few but specific | many and diffuse |
| Focus | communication | cognitive, social, neuropsychological |

their child's future. This vision is a crucial factor in communication counseling, because it introduces a new player at the table, as it were. Although no literature directly addresses this issue, counseling parents concerning "the child who might have been" appears to be different in some ways from counseling them about "the child who used to be." That is, the experience that parents have had with their previously normal child may modify their counseling needs.

This perspective of loss is important for the communication counselor working with these families, as well as an awareness that parents' emotions such as disappointment, anger, frustration, and resentment may accompany these later-occurring disorders in greater degrees than for the early-onset disorders. Also, these parents have not lived and had the chance to grow with their child's problems in the foreground, as have parents of at-risk children (such as Jacob's father, Cynthia Kidder, and Sue Swenson, as described in Chapter 4). Rather, they have had a period, even if only a brief one, of enjoying the normal development that preceded onset of their child's communication problems. The contrast they subsequently experience may have persistent effects.

Parents of stuttering and TBI children may possibly learn much from the parents of children whose problems came earlier, the veterans. For example, parents of children with Down syndrome or severe hearing losses have had experiences that may benefit parents who have much more limited exposure to the kinds of problems involved. Parents of children with early-onset disorders also may be better grounded, because they are further along in acknowledging and accepting their children's differences.

Family expectations concerning how their children will turn out is a topic of considerable complexity and controversy in the mental health literature, and largely beyond our scope of practice. Nevertheless, parental expectations are likely to have unique repercussions when a previously normally developing child incurs a physical, cognitive, or communication disorder or some combination of such disorders. It is possible that the longer parents have experienced a child's normal development, the more difficult it is for them to cope with the changed reality. Thus, it is a possibility that Down syndrome may in some way be easier for parents to accept than stuttering, and early TBI may be less devastating for families than late TBI. This possibility may merit formal clinical study; in any case, the timing factor is a significant counseling issue.

Another aspect of the delay in onset is that SLP-As often are the professionals who break the news, at least in relation to stuttering and SLI, or possibly confirm what parents have already figured out. Pediatricians typically have little information on normal language development, and although they often refer families to SLP-As, they generally do not prepare parents for the results of SLP-A assessments. Breaking the news itself calls for counseling skill.

## What Are the Outcomes?

Will Kenny, a very early stutterer, be among the 80% of stuttering children who become normal speakers? Or will his stuttering continue despite therapy and be an influential factor in his adult life? Will Janet, who has SLI, become a normal language user? Or will she remain challenged by language and learning disabilities (LLD) throughout her life? With TBI, what are the long-term consequences, not only for Barry, who has a severe head injury, but also for Barbra, whose head injury was comparatively mild? Will Barry ever be able to manage on his own? Or will he always be dependent on others to survive? Will Barbra be able to complete high school or go to college?

Worrying about the future is the major ingredient of anxiety, and forecasting outcomes for disorders such as these is a tricky and difficult business. These disorders have murky outcomes and unclear causes, and their deviations from the expected course created by previous normalcy make the counseling issues they raise at least as challenging as those encountered in counseling parents of children who are at risk almost from the time of their birth. The need for optimism and resilience is at least as high. For children and families whose problems are skewed toward the severe end of each disorder's continuum, resilience and optimism may be difficult to achieve.

## Severity

For both TBI and stuttering, there is a wide range of severity. High school football players experiencing a single concussion probably are not in need of much clinical intervention, or of communication counseling. Nor are preschool children whose stuttering is extremely mild, unless it worsens over time. Few such children, however, come to the attention of SLP-As in the first place. SLP-As are more likely to have clinical relationships with affected children whose problems are moderate or severe. Nonetheless, it is worth noting that severity and the extent of need for counseling are not necessarily correlated. This seems particularly relevant for so-called *covert stuttering*, in which the observable aspects of stuttering have disappeared but the dread of speaking remains.

Symptom severity creates an interesting and challenging dilemma for counselors. Consider, for example, a group of parents of adolescents with TBI. What happens if both Barry's and Barbra's parents attend the same support group? Barbra's family is concerned with school reintegration, whereas Barry's parents wonder if their son can ever successfully integrate into a group home. It seems logical to form groups on the basis of diagnosis. So long as parents of children whose disorders are going to worsen are not mixed with parents of those who are likely to improve, however, a better solution often is to form parent groups based on issues of severity, regardless of etiology. Symptom severity also is an issue that supports the need for individual parental counseling.

## Focus Disorders and Their Differences

In addition to similarities, children and families with TBI and stuttering also have differences that affect counseling. Disorders such as SLI and voice may share some problems with either TBI or stuttering. Some of the important differences are discussed next.

### Etiology

Most of the disorders described in Chapter 4 have relatively clear causes, or they share relatively clear-cut characteristics that permit parents to come to some understanding of what brought about the disorder. Such is not the case with the disorders discussed in this chapter. Although it is the focus of current genetic research, the cause of stuttering (and SLI) is not yet known. Whether stuttering results from subtle brain damage such as the presence of extra gyri or decreased fiber tracts as documented in some adults who stutter (Foundas, Bollich, Cory, Hurley, & Heilman, 2001; Sommer, Koch, Paulus, Weiller, & Buchel, 2002), genetic factors, some environmental determinants, or a combination of some or all of these factors has been debated for longer than 50 years, and the issue remains unresolved. For stuttering (and for SLI and phonological disorders), we have few satisfactory answers to parents' enduring questions such as "How did this happen?" or "Why did this happen?" This situation provides another instance in which counselors must learn to say "I don't know" in a variety of principled ways and to be particularly sensitive to the effects of having to say it.

By contrast, TBI results from car crashes, falls, and other accidents that cause brain damage. This damage typically is widespread and hard to visualize by imaging techniques in terms of extent and severity. The fact that TBI brains often "look normal" complicates the ability of health care professionals to give cogent information. Unfortunately, diffuse damage limits the likelihood that professionals can predict the specific problems that can result. Diffuse brain damage common in TBI produces a range of behavioral outcomes, creating perplexing agendas for communication counseling. Nevertheless, with assistance, most families can achieve good understanding of what has caused the problems.

## Fluctuations and Variability

SLP-As are required to demonstrate their tolerance for variability almost every day. Disorders of human communication share a propensity for individual variation, as well as day-to-day fluctuation in the same person. However, variability is particularly marked in stuttering. For example, affected children whose stuttering usually is severe may have occasional days of near-perfect fluency and days that are awful. The fluent good days may serve as painful reminders to parents of "the child who used to be"—already mentioned as a counseling concern of significance. Regardless, counselors have a role to play in helping parents and children to determine what triggers both the fluent and the nonfluent days. The goal is to capitalize on what can be learned (from the good days) and what should be avoided (from the bad ones).

## Concomitant Problems

Stuttering comes with relatively extensive emotional baggage, as discussed later in the chapter. A substantial number of stuttering children also are thought to have accompanying phonological and possibly language-learning problems. Stuttering does not protect the affected person from other communication disorders. But the emotional accompaniments of stuttering represent the largest concerns in communication counseling.

In marked contrast, TBI may be associated with a vast range of concomitant problems, extending from cognitive and neuropsychological issues, to emotional, educational, and psychosocial ones. When any of this array of problems affects a particular brain-injured child and his or her family, it plays a major role in counseling. Problems associated with TBI also are discussed in more detail later in this chapter.

## Counseling Responsibilities

The concomitant problems in large measure determine the focus of counseling efforts with many children who have late-developing disorders of communication. Stuttering, SLI, and phonological disorders and, to some extent, voice disorders in children are centered clinically in the discipline of human communication disorders. They share this feature with hearing impairment and maxillofacial disorders in children, as described in Chapter 4. The broad education of such children is not focused in communication, but it puts their counseling there. Such heightened focus on communication is another reason why counselors in this profession often are messengers who bring the bad news to many families of such children.

By contrast, the counseling focus for TBI is considerably more encompassing and typically requires the services of a multidisciplinary team. SLP-As certainly function as members of such a team, but the primary counseling role may be played by any of a variety of team members, including social workers, neuropsychologists, or other rehabilitation specialists. This also is the case with many children affected by the disorders covered in Chapter 4—those on the autism spectrum and those with mental retardation and other neurological disorders.

# Listening to the Stories

Stories are clinically as relevant for parents of children with these late-appearing problems as it is are for those of early-appearing ones. Older children and adolescents also have their own stories to tell. The basic reasons for encouraging stories remain the same, but with additional urgencies. One is that parents of children with these disorders appear to have more limited access to self-help resources and websites[1] where they can experience the stories of others and potentially learn from them or be positively influenced by them. For example, parents of children with SLI will find stories of children similar to theirs only in more general works on communication on disorders in childhood. Because self-help books thrive on stories, and because telling one's stories and listening to others' stories have healing power, it is unfortunate that this literature is relatively sparse. This lack may be related to the issues raised earlier about uncertainty of what the future holds, coupled with the disappointment of losing, in some sense, the child who was free of these disorders.

The circumstances surrounding their children's communication problems may make it more difficult for parents to be resilient and optimistic. If such is the case, it raises new challenges in communication counseling, possibly even new "ghosts" in the therapy room, in addition to the ones talked about in Chapter 4. The communication counselor must not limit story seeking to only the "bad stuff." To maximize the positive and explore and shape resilience and optimism, stories about what is going well are at least as important as the painful ones.

Thus, encouraging parents of children with late-developing problems to tell their stories is imperative; as mentioned previously, the stimulus for story-telling is simply to ask to hear them. In assessment and in subsequent individual sessions, counselors need to identify the disorienting dilemmas and recognize the opportunities they provide for growth and change. In parent groups, the story-telling process presents opportunities to learn from others as well.

---

[1]Some particularly relevant websites are listed at the end of the chapter.

## What are Parents' Worries?

The major issues discussed in Chapter 4 all are applicable and need not be repeated here. Nevertheless, certain issues may be more important with some disorders than with others. For example, the parents of Sam, who stutters, may be relatively unconcerned about issues of independence, because there are many examples of people who have overcome stuttering, as well as of successful people who continue to stutter. Instead, Sam's parents may settle their anxieties and worries on the cascade of social consequences that could leave Sam with a limited circle of friends when he grows up. By contrast, Miles has had a severe head injury. His parents also may worry about acceptance but are concerned about safety, independence, and happiness as well. Because of its severity, Miles' problem is linked to the broader concerns of parents from Chapter 4.

The smaller worries also are much the same as those described in Chapter 4 except that those for toddlers have been replaced by worries about school and peer relationships. The concerns listed in Box 5.2 can be added to those listed in Boxes 4.3 and 4.4. Counselors may find it useful to try out different answers to relevant questions from parents, to prepare for when such questions are asked in clinical practice.

"Counseling moments," before or after sessions, continue to arise. Now many of the questions, however, come not only from parents but also from the affected children themselves. Box 5.3 contains a sampling of such questions.

---

### Box 5.2 Parent Worries for
### Older Children with Communication Disorders

- Lack of friends at school
- How to increase inclusion
- How to manage teasing
- Making school a more positive experience

## Box 5.3 "Counseling Moments" with Parents and Children with Later-Developing Communication Disorders

As in Chapter 4, a "counseling moment" and its response constitutes something that is not within your scope of practice. If you feel it is not, then answer from that perspective. If you decide it is within your scope of practice, answer from the latter perspective. More than one answer probably is warranted for most of the "moments."

### Parents' Moments

"I don't know what to do when Lindy says the kids laugh at her in school."

"It kills me that Eric has no friends. How can we get other kids to realize that just because he sounds funny and looks kind of different, he's a really swell little guy?"

"I've heard from my neighbor that glucosamine is effective in reducing stuttering. Can you send us to a website that has more information on this?"

"If we get her an AAC device, will it help her to talk, or will she just give up trying?"

"It's really getting worse every day. I hardly sleep, I am losing weight, I have no energy or ambition, and I am wondering if it's worth it to keep on trying . . . "

"I've tried to explain to his teacher that Mark needs more time and patience than the other kids. I don't think she's ever had to deal with an Asperger's kid in her classroom before. I don't know what to do."

"Since his TBI, just about all his friends have deserted him. He hates being back in school and being ignored. I even tried to pay one of the girls in his old gang to go to the movies with him, and she refused. I don't know what to do."

> **Children's Moments**
>
> "Look, I'm 13 years old and I want to make my own decisions about therapy. Mom says she agrees, but I live with Grandpa and Grandma, and they want me to keep coming. What do you think?
>
> "Why do I stutter?"
>
> "I don't have any friends. I am very sad."
>
> "Why do I have to wear this stupid big old hearing aid?"
>
> "I'm the only kid in the whole class who has to go to therapy! That's not fair—lotsa kids in there talk funny!"

The vital importance of the technical skill of listening bears reemphasizing here. Fred Rogers (2003) said it simply and well:

> In times of stress, the best thing we can do for each other is to listen with our ears and with our hearts and to be assured that our questions are just as important as our answers (p. 79).

## Unique Features of the Counseling Process for Stuttering and TBI

First for stuttering and then for TBI, this section addresses the same issues covered in Chapter 4 for those focus disorders—namely, cause, course, accompanying problems, and sources of help. Many features of these two disorders are shared by other communication problems.

### Stuttering

Over decades of teaching survey courses in speech pathology, I have been consistently impressed with the power of the relatively infrequently occurring disorder of stuttering to draw students deeply into the subject of human communication and its disorders. Perceived by most beginners as our discipline's most exotic problem, stuttering's lure perhaps comes from the uncertainties of its cause and its course, and the effects both on those who stutter and on their families. The counseling issues that surround cause and course are discussed first.

## Cause

Stuttering most likely results from a constellation of predispositional factors not yet known, and in proportions that are unclear as well. Genetic and neurologic features probably play a role, along with dynamic environmental and psycholinguistic features that are in and of themselves each insufficient to explain the phenomenon. Hypotheses about stuttering abound, and most of them have accompanying treatment implications. Bennett (2006) discusses at least 10 such instantiations in her recent text. Skilled communication counselors who work with stuttering children and families need to be aware of their own biases concerning the etiology of stuttering. Furthermore, counselors have a responsibility to communicate those biases as clearly as they can to the families with whom they work. Box 5.4 lists ALH's biases, by way of example.

Both the lay and the professional literature on stuttering stress the importance of dealing with the potential of parental guilt concerning stuttering. That guilt is so prominently featured in stuttering work is likely to be due to the foggy and conjectural nature of cause. Communication counselors who work with stutterers and their families must be highly sensitive to this issue and must make it very clear that it is not within parents' power to create stuttering in their children—that although whatever the etiological "stew" consists of is unclear, it certainly has more than one ingredient.

## Course

Almost equally baffling is the course of the disorder. A majority of children who come to the early attention of SLPs recover normal speech spontaneously; others require therapy to recover. Some grow to adulthood still stuttering. Even some who have had superb therapy continue to stutter throughout their lives. Who is to tell

## Box 5.4 Addressing a Tough Question: What Causes Stuttering?

The following parent–communication counselor dialogue, from my own clinical experience, is presented as a possible model for how to discuss the etiology of stuttering.

PARENT: Why does Billy stutter? What causes stuttering?

CLINICIAN: I'll answer this, but only if you will share with me your reactions to my answer, and tell me what you think causes it. Okay?

PARENT: Fair enough.

CLINICIAN: Well, I need to start by admitting that I don't truly know—no one's come up with a simple answer yet. I *suspect* that a whole bunch of little, hard-to-find factors bring it about, but this is only a guess. As I've mentioned, the focus of my work has always been on brain and language, so that my bias is that in stuttering there is some kind of unusual brain wiring that is the trigger, but it takes a lot of other influences as well to pull the trigger. I want to go on, but before I do, I hope you understand that I don't believe this "brain problem" is very serious in and of itself. It is a brain difference, not much else. Am I being clear?

PARENT: Kinda. You're not saying that Billy has really bad brain damage?

CLINICIAN: No-no-no. I am only saying that his brain wiring is probably a trigger. You know he is an okay kid in the big picture of doing his schoolwork and stuff, right? And even his periods of fluency would give us a notion that this is not big-deal brain damage.

PARENT: Got it. So what does the brain trigger off that makes Billy stutter?

CLINICIAN: Here is where I go mushy: I don't know. Perhaps it is his sensitivity to how he sounds, or how other people react, or his interpretation of how other kids always speak smoothly. (This is not true, of course—they have bumpy speech, too, but I suspect Billy never notices *that*!) Maybe it is buried in his genes, but that's no real explanation either. By the way, what I don't think that just because we can't say that this or that is the cause, we can't be helpful. We don't know the causes of a lot of stuff. We need to move on from "why it is, to what would help? Okay—end of lecture, almost. But *you* did not cause Billy to stutter. You are just not that powerful! A lot of stuff came together to make that happen. Now it's *your* turn.

the difference at stuttering's onset and how is it to be told? Issues concerning even the early course of stuttering are controversial. For example, following diagnosis, some authorities (e.g., Curlee & Yairi, 1997) recommend waiting for a period of time to pass before beginning direct intervention, while families try to become more focused listeners, and to take speaking and environmental pressure away from their young stutterer. The goal of this approach is to engage parents in behaviors that may facilitate spontaneous recovery. Other authorities (Ingham & Cordes, 1998) urge early intervention, making the case that even if spontaneous recovery occurs, early intervention, being benign, will do no harm. Proponents on either side of this issue can bring data to bear on the correctness of their positions. This can only be baffling to parents and give rise to another counseling concern: Is "the child that was" permanently lost or only mislaid? In the face of such uncertainty, how can plans be made?

Of note, possibly the most successful management program currently available for children who stutter is the Lidcombe Program (Onslow and Packman, 1999) Onslow, 2003, Onslow, Packman, & Harrison, 2003). Data from this program, which are available for more than 250 children, indicate that intervention begun early is the most effective (Jones et al., 2005). Although the database is impressive, many unresolved issues remain (see Ratner, 2005, Bernstein Ratner & Guitar, 2006, ). (For example, what proportion of the 80% of children who recover are in the database?) Nevertheless, timing of intervention does seem to be of the essence, and many of the suggestions in this chapter are for children who are still stuttering by the time they reach kindergarten or grade school or later.

## *Problems Accompanying Stuttering*

The problems that accompany stuttering are monumental, although fortunately they are relatively few in number. Most approaches to stuttering are balanced attempts both to modify stuttered speech and to deal with its negative psychological consequences. Depending on particular events, the scales may be tipped either to stuttering's audible aspects or to its accompanying problems. In either case, remediation of stuttering has emphasized counseling more than is true for most other speech, hearing, or language disorders.

Sheehan coined the metaphor "Iceberg of Stuttering," with stuttering behavior itself representing only the tip (Sheehan, 1970). Underneath this stuttering iceberg lurk (in order, on the way down into the depths) fear, shame, guilt, anxiety, hopelessness, isolation, and denial.[2] One of the questionable implications of this metaphor is that stuttered speech behavior is presented as small relative to the bigger underlying issues. Nevertheless, the metaphor, originally referring to stuttering in adults, illustrates Sheehan's belief that the overt behavior of stuttering probably is not manageable without some attention being paid to the accompanying (or possibly under-lying) psychodynamics.

If true, the model also is relevant to counseling children who are beginning to stutter. It seems likely that the superficial charac-teristics of dysfluency probably occur first, with the underliers being learned only with repeated negative experiences (a point in favor of early intervention), and probably in some semblance of Sheehan's order; fear of talking clearly precedes some of the other more difficult-to-operationalize dimensions. Thus, one of the early responsibilities of communication counselors is to help parents (and, depending on their age, children directly) capitalize on or help the stuttering child to develop age-appropriate versions of character strengths such as bravery, humor, and social intelligence and, addi-tionally, resilience. The point of such work should be to forestall fear and to avert the downward slide into shame, anxiety, hopeless-ness, and the rest. Box 5.5 provides some examples of how this may be done with parents.

---

[2]For a clear explication and a dynamic understanding of Sheehan's "iceberg" and its relationship to stuttering, visit the website of Russ Hicks, listed at the end of the chapter.

**Box 5.5  Promoting the Positive for
Parents of Stuttering Children**

■ Ask parents to set aside time (dinnertime probably is best) once a week to discuss the good things that happened to the child this week, and what *he* or *she* did to bring them about. Everyone has to participate, parents too, to set the examples and rules. They don't have to be big things (although they can be): for example, for the child, finally saving enough of his or her allowance to buy a big chocolate ice cream cone, or for Mom, finally making time to get a massage, or for Dad, going on a hike on Sunday. Then move this schedule from weekly to daily—possibly sharing the events at bedtime. For older children, it is fun to write them on cards and then pull the cards from a hat for discussion.

■ Ask parents to take the VIA and identify their five signature strengths. Older kids can take the child version, or the clinician can help them to identify their strengths using the list in Chapter 2. Ask both parents and kids to tell a story about how they used their strengths. Ask them to use a strength in a new way each week, and discuss it at home. This should not be merely a recital for kids—parents need to participate too.

■ Another weekly activity could involve gratitude. Tell the child to think of a person (or pet) who was very nice to him or her this week. What did the person do? Did the child remember to say thank you? If not, the child can be encouraged to thank the person at their next encounter.

■ Ask parents to write a paragraph about their stuttering child at his or her best. Ask them to write another statement about them at their best with their stuttering child. What strengths does this reveal?

■ Finally, a suggestion from my colleague Noel Matkin, PhD (personal communication, 2006): Dr. Matkin pointed out that one of the most productive ways to promote school inclusion of deaf and hearing-impaired children is for parents to be on the alert for and to foster and nurture talent or interest in sports. That needs to be expanded to children with communication disorders of all kinds, and to other activities such as playing musical instruments or getting involved in dance or drama.

Children may not end up playing professional basketball or swimming on a local swimming team; they may not end up performing in a big symphony orchestra or designing sets for Broadway plays. But they might. And even if they don't, they might have a grand time at the Special Olympics! The important thing is to be part of a group with a shared, cohesive agenda.

## Sources of Family Support

Listed at the end of the chapter are websites that may be useful for parents of children who are potential stutterers, as well as those who develop into stutterers. Communication counselors are urged to study them carefully. Many of these sources focus on what is wrong, rather than taking a more positive view. With the exception of enthusiastic and positive cheerleading from stuttering individuals such as Russ Hicks and from the National Stuttering Association, the overwhelming bias is negative, resulting in problem-focused rather than solution-focused agendas. The intrinsic contradictions built into the management of stuttering, along with a sort of obeisance to the power of "experts" (professionals) in its management, probably are the cause. Box 5.6 lists some of the contradictions that require discussion and probably resolution, for counseling to be effective.

The huge concern about the speaking environments of stuttering children is puzzling, when (for example) the speaking environments of children with cleft lip and palate are, by comparison, relatively unexplored. Their circumstances should be relatively similar—after all, children with many maxillofacial abnormalities also seem likely candidates for teasing. Do peers have a harder time accepting communication differences when they are unaccompanied by obvious physical differences? The negative reaction may be based in part on stuttering's variability—that is, do "normal" chil-

---

**Box 5.6 Contradictions: Considerations
in Counseling for Stutterers and Their Families**

I need to acknowledge stuttering and believe it is okay for
me to stutter—no big deal.

*versus*

I must be a fluent speaker.

When my speech is normal, I will be accepted.

*versus*

We are more than the way we talk.

Fluent speech

*versus*

Compensatory strategies

I should not pay attention to my child's dysfluencies.

*versus*

I use a notebook to record the circumstances when my child
is fluent and dysfluent.

---

dren perceive the child who stutters only intermittently as just
shamming? The combination of physical and communication differences may in essence force children who have both disorders to
learn to cast off ridicule more easily, so that they ending up with
kind of peculiar advantage. Perhaps children who live with maxillofacial anomalies may simply have learned to be tougher. The support of their parents may also have played a role. Finally,
a crucial factor in the difference between the experiences of these
children and those who stutter probably is the late arrival of the
bad news in the case of stuttering and the need for parents to
reassess expectations.[3]

Finally, it is important to take into account the issue of expertise,
raised in Chapter 1. For stuttering, more than for many other communication disorders, "experts" appear to be defined specifically as

---

[3]A useful handbook on teasing is *Bullying and Teasing: Helping Children Who
Stutter* by Yaruss, Murphy, Quesal, and Reardon (2004). Although addressed to
stuttering children, it has implications for other communication disorders as well.

researchers and clinicians whose focus has been on understanding all there is to understand about stuttering from an outsider's perspective. This may well be related to the powerful influence of professionals who themselves were stutterers, such as Wendell Johnson and Charles Van Riper, on the development of speech pathology and on clinicians' specific role in stuttering management. These professionals had the credibility of both being inside experts and outside experts on top of that. The tradition of stuttering professional experts, functioning as researchers, clinicians, role models, and people who experience the problem firsthand flourished through the work of Dean Williams, Hugo Gregory, and others and persists today. The contributions of such individuals are undeniable—but they may inadvertently have made it harder to find the shared expertise provided by stuttering children and their families who did not choose a professional path. Because so little is understood about stuttering, counseling may be more helpful if family and stuttering children and adults are recognized fully as expert stakeholders.

One reason for the Lidcombe Program's success may be due to this explicit involvement of families and their empowerment in the management of their child's stuttering. Families are recognized as having the "insider perspective," and they are expected to act from this perspective. In fact, the supervising clinician respects and encourages family input in planning the teaching experiences they are expected to provide. Furthermore, parental observation and evaluation probably play major roles in success or failure using the Lidcombe approach.[4] If this is the case, the implications for counseling are clear. Some comments on the Lidcombe approach, from the standpoint of positive psychology, are presented in Box 5.7.

## Traumatic Brain Injury

TBI lacks stuttering's inherent "singleness" of causation, course, and other features. Because brain damage itself may affect different brain regions and result in both local and more global effects, and because it can vary extremely in its effects, TBI provides an interesting counterpoint to stuttering. It also presents different counseling challenges.

---

[4]For a description of how parents can participate in developing the teaching experiences, see Bernstein Ratner and Guitar's (2006) comprehensive text on stuttering.

---

### Box 5.7 Lidcombe and Positive Psychology

In Chapter 2, Frederickson and Losada* (2005) suggested that a positive dynamic relationship between positive and negative comments for enhancing adult interactions requires a ratio of 3:1—three positive comments for every negative comment, with a maximum ratio of 12:1. Lidcombe suggests a 5:1 ratio —five positive comments for each "corrective" response to stuttering. For kids in trouble, this proportion seems a bit thin; a 7:1 ratio is more likely to provide maximal benefit.

In Chapter 3, Gable and colleagues[†] showed that only active constructive responding fosters positive relationships. ("Uh-huh" responses don't count!) Parents' "corrective" responses to stuttering children should be "constructive" as well.

---

*Frederickson, B. L., & Losada, M. (2005). Positive affect and the complex dynamics of human flourishing. *American Psychologist, 60,* 687–686.

[†]Gable, S., Reis, H., Impett, E., & Asher, E. (2004). What do you do when things go right? The intrapersonal and interpersonal benefits of sharing good events. *Journal of Personality and Social Psychology, 87,* 228–245.

---

### Causes

The causes of TBI generally are clear. With events that result in injuries to the head, and therefore to the brain, such as motor vehicle accidents, falls, and a host of other accidents such as partial drowning, the cause of the traumatic injury usually is easy to trace and not particularly mysterious. Thus, it is not the cause of the injury per se that is a significant counseling issue. Rather, it is the effects of that injury to a particular individual. Communication counselors who work with people who have incurred focal brain injury (such as that due to strokes in adults or children), as well as their families, recognize the difficulties in helping them to understand these physiologically relatively simpler problems. In the case of TBI, the informational burden for clinicians is even greater. However, one general principle for these neurogenic disorders is that the less the extent of brain damage, the greater the chances for recovery.

Clarity of cause can be a double-edged sword, particularly in relation to childhood TBI. If Eddie's TBI is the result of a motor vehicle accident that occurred while his father Joe was driving, it probably is hard for Joe to take the word "accident" at face value, and to escape feelings of responsibility and possibly guilt for Eddie's problems. If Sally, Eddie's mother, also was in the car and had forgotten to ensure that Eddie's seat belt was fastened, she may experience similar feelings. Issues such as these considerably cloud the counseling picture and in many cases extend beyond the professional talents and responsibilities of communication counselors. It is mandatory for counselors to be alert, aware, observant, and ready with a list of referrals to more appropriate specialists.

The "accident" implicit in many TBI cases brings another set of counseling concerns in relation to possible litigation. It is an issue even in instances with little contentiousness or animosity and in which a sense of fairness guides parents to seek compensation for the loss of "the child who was," or of the child's ability to live the life expected before the TBI. Parents may have difficulty in maintaining balance or may have mixed feelings about restitution or resolution. Make no mistake: the vast majority of TBI parents of a child who has sustained a TBI would give up litigation in a flash if their injured child could be returned to them as before the accident. The point is merely that litigation may complicate counseling.

### *Course*

Neuroplasticity is a major factor in the process of recovery from TBI. Our understanding of neuroplasticity has greatly increased over the past decade. We now recognize that plasticity is a characteristic not simply of the younger brain but of the brain itself—possibly across the lifespan. Nevertheless younger brains fare much better (i.e., demonstrate greater plasticity) than do older ones.

Even so, the course of recovery from TBI is extremely difficult to predict. One clue comes from duration of coma in cases of TBI that result in a prolonged period of unconsciousness. As a rule, the longer the period of coma, the less likely full recovery is. For milder injuries, such as concussion, the effects of TBI may be transitory, but repeated concussion increases the likelihood of permanent damage. Although few communication counselors are likely to be involved with comatose children, clinicians who work in acute care settings sometimes encounter parents at bedside. During this time, parents are likely to be in shock or, when the coma is prolonged, beginning an uneasy acknowledgment. In this situation, the counselor should focus on accepting parents' feelings at that time, and not on handing out information about what to expect, or guessing about outcomes. The counselor simply does not know and should be honest about saying so.

This picture changes when children and adolescents do indeed begin measurable recovery. Spontaneous recovery from TBI in children is a stepwise and unpredictable process, lacking the smoother, negatively accelerated features of adult recovery from stroke. This is the first factor that makes TBI outcome unpredictable. In addition, for a substantial number of children and adolescents, recovery may appear to be complete following extensive rehabilitation in a nurturing supportive environment, but profound problems may become evident when they return to the hustle and bustle of everyday life.

Children may be particularly affected when they return to their former schools and begin to interact with their classmates again. This is a major reason why Ylvisaker and Feeney (1998) insist on the importance of involving and training everyday people in the lives of persons with TBI. There are other reasons as well, which follow largely from the scope of problems likely to be associated with TBI.

### Accompanying Problems

SLP-As are aware that the communication of children and adolescents with TBI may very likely come embedded in a distressingly broad range of cognitive, emotional, and psychosocial and physical problems. From a counseling perspective, the most debilitating are likely to be those associated with the frontal lobe dysfunctions that occur frequently in TBI, and with the impairments in systems and processes of cognition that are likely to be its concomitants. Ylvisaker and Feeney (1998) provide a comprehensive listing. For frontal lobe dysfunction, these include lack of self-awareness of strengths and weaknesses; difficulty in goal-setting, planning, and organizing; difficulties in both initiating and inhibiting behaviors; and problems in self-monitoring and self-evaluating, problem-solving, and strategic thinking.

For cognitive components, Ylvisaker and Feeny (1998) list most forms of memory, including short- and long-term memory and working memory; prospective memory also should be included.

These investigators also list the component processes of attention, perception, new learning, organization, and reasoning. Normal cognitive functioning includes all of these components and processes, which are highly interrelated. Although they may not all be affected in TBI, the possibility nonetheless exists. Furthermore, in some children and adolescents (depending on age at onset), specific processes may fail to develop adequately. All are targets of direct service and also complicate communication counseling.

In many instances, communication counselors are likely to see manifestations such cognitive problems, rather than purely linguistic consequences. This constellation of head-injury accompaniments increases the likelihood that the child with TBI also will have psychosocial problems. In some children and adolescents, difficulties can arise with peer relationships. Thus, helping brain-injured children to develop the necessary functional and social skills for such relationships may constitute a substantial piece of the counseling picture.

For all of these reasons, it seems crucial for SLP-As to function as members of an interdisciplinary team for the management of TBI. Because TBI rehabilitation teams in urban rehabilitation settings typically include psychologists, neuropsychologists, and social workers, a team approach is not particularly difficult to achieve in such cases. In more rural settings, however, where rehabilitation for persons with milder head injuries may be less well organized and involve fewer specialists, public school personnel may be required to substitute for an interdisciplinary team. Thus, SLP-As' counseling responsibilities with TBI may vary widely. Nevertheless, the central issues often have more to do with the "alongside problems" than with the effects of communication disorders specifically.

### Helping with the Alongside Problems

The "alongside problems" again raise the question of expertise. As noted, plenty of professional experts are on most TBI children's teams. But what about the "insider views"? Children with new TBIs probably will need to be guided into a new and altered expertise; they must live with their injuries at least for a while before they can be reliable observers of their own behavior. One counseling responsibility is to help them develop this skill.

The family is another matter. When their children have more severe TBIs, parents are in the best position to help the other experts to connect the brain-injured child with the one they knew before. To counsel families appropriately, clinicians often are dependent on family expertise. But this is a difficult situation, if not a slippery slope: Guiding parents to inform you about their child as he or she used to be, while simultaneously broadcasting the message that this child has now changed, requires sensitivity

In Chapter 7, the concept of ambiguous loss (Boss, 1999) is explored in detail in relation to adults with disorders of downward progression. Readers are forewarned that families of both children and adults with TBI also potentially face the issue of what Boss calls "saying goodbye without leaving." The frequently heard poignant comment that the child, adolescent, or adult with TBI is a "different person" reflects this notion. Thus, many of the issues discussed in Chapter 7 apply to TBI as well.

Finally, many rehabilitation models exist for children and adults who have incurred TBI. It is not in the purview of this book to endorse one model over another. However, from a counseling perspective, the most powerful models are those that from the beginning incorporate what Ylvisaker and Feeney (1998) term the *everyday* (that is, everyday people, everyday settings, and everyday routines). The goal of all of the direct work, as well as the counseling related to this approach, is societal reintegration. Ylvisaker and Feeney stress ways to compensate for frontal lobe dysfunction, along with the other cognitive problems, and define ways to get on with life through self-talk and self-coaching, developing compensatory routines, reestablishing social skills, finding new ways to plan that take TBI into account, and so forth. Thus, at its core, their approach is a form of counseling/coaching.

### Sources of Family Support

Listed at the end of the chapter is a sampling of websites for TBI, with links that can direct the family researcher to reach a broader selection. Again, support groups are readily accessible, particularly through www.biausa.org. As with stuttering, however, positive and forward-looking comments are lacking. With TBI, the website's emphasis on young adults, who truly dominate the age-at-onset statistics, may account for this lack. According to the NIH, although more than 1 million children each year incur head injuries, "only" 30,000 of them incur significant brain injury as a result. The incidence of TBI is highest in the United States for young people 15 to 24 years of age. But late onset also plays a role, as parents (and older children) face altered and more modest expectations and the abundant resources and support needed to manage associated problems are lacking.

## Some Limitations to Current Approaches to Counseling Children

As noted, SLPs who work with clients who stutter and with those who have incurred TBI (across the age span) and their families have specifically and consistently addressed their counseling responsibilities for a number of years. Only clinicians who work with voice disorders seem to be as committed to counseling for their clients. However, psychotherapeutic principles have served as the model for this work; accordingly, counseling has been concerned primarily with helping clients and their families to understand the causes and dynamics of their disorders and, essentially, "what is wrong." Typically these issues are prerequisites, or co-requisites, to changing and moving on. Thus, in coupling them with techniques for increasing fluent speech, SLPs risk creating contradictions that may undermine the counseling process. Box 5.6 listed some contradictions that illustrate this point in relation to stuttering.

The issue of acknowledgment of stuttering is used as an example here. For most children and adults who stutter, acceptance of their stuttering is a piece of their counseling mantra. But coupling acceptance with the need to change the accepted behavior sends a mixed message: "Stuttering is the result of some unknown combination of known factors that influence my life, yet I must do the best that I can, despite these mysterious and frightening factors, to make my speech normal."

Not only is this message contradictory, but it also assumes that stuttering is something to be "gotten over." Positive psychology can help affected persons (both children and adults and their families) to deal with the difficulty of simply changing behavior. If the goal is to speak more fluently (and there is evidence to support the effectiveness of treatment to help achieve this goal), then perhaps it would be prudent for SLPs to assist their clients to develop skills, such as resilience, that can help them meet the challenges inherent in making those changes. It seems clear that people who stutter are frustrated by their inability to control their speech mechanism, and they want to speak more fluently. In fact, they know what fluent speech can be like because they have periods of fluent, seemingly normal speech.

In parallel with Seligman's concept (2002) that the opposite of depression is not happiness but simply "not depressed," the opposite of stuttering is not perfect speech (and, by extension, a perfect life) but just "not stuttering." Coaching and counseling stemming from a positive psychology perspective use self-examination and exercises designed to incorporate the science of happiness into living an authentically happier life. A positive psychological perspective on communication counseling would have counselors work with individuals with communication problems do something similar.

A good example stems from the Lidcombe approach (Onslow, Packman & Harrison, 2003) to stuttering mentioned earlier. Contrary to traditional approaches that counsel parents to downplay dysfluency, Lidcome encourages them play an active role in acknowledging and helping their child to do something about the dysfluencies. They are encouraged to give their children practical advice, rather than the ubiquitous "relax and slow down," which may or may not be helpful. Bernstein Ratner and Guitar (2006) observe that by paying attention to their child's dysfluencies in this way, parents may actually help to normalize the child's speech.

## The Wellness Perspective

The wellness perspective is offered as a balance to more traditional approaches, because it avoids the inherent contradictions between "accept it" and "change it." A wellness perspective is an attempt to move beyond the "Popeye approach"—that is, "I am what I am, a stutterer. I have to learn to live with it, and you must accept me as I am." A wellness perspective is more akin to the following: "For me, stuttering just *is*. I will change what I can and learn to live with what I cannot. I need to move on, beyond an identity as just someone who stutters."

Because of the anxiety factor, stuttering in adults has previously been mentioned as perhaps an appropriate area for intervention by cognitive-behavioral therapy (CBT) techniques, which, as you may recall, are at least grandparents to the positive psychology movement. Ratner (2005) noted that CBT has been successfully used to treat "communicative anxiety" and "to combat speaking fears and anxieties in stuttering." A recent study by Klein and Amster (2005) used CBT to treat stuttering adults who were also perfectionists. Their results were promising, including well-maintained decrements in both stuttering and perfectionism. Furthermore, according to the website (www3.fhs.usyd.edu.au/asrcwww/treatment/lidcombe.htm) for the Lidcombe Center, CBT currently is the subject of research that incorporates it into "standard" therapy for adults who stutter. This suggests one way in which wellness perspectives can influence the treatment of stuttering.

The case for TBI is somewhat similar, but not identical. Stuttering children may make their stuttering the scapegoat for some or all of their other problems. By contrast, children with TBI are likely to be anosognosic and fail to recognize their problems; this makes realizing and accepting their TBI-associated limitations an important initial goal. Another crucial difference is in the optimal self-management approach with TBI, outlined as follows: "Learn what you need to do, and what supports what you need to do. Change what you can. Find strategies and practice strategies that work. Move on." Self-efficacy, always important, is crucial here.

## Some Direct Resilience and Change Techniques

An important component of counseling with stuttering and TBI is training in resilience and change—in how to move on and become tough and optimistic, with greater capacity for happiness. The techniques presented here are specific for stuttering but are equally applicable to TBI and to many of the other problems that occur as counseling issues later in childhood. They also can be used with children with the focus disorders described in Chapter 4, as they grow older. Some of these ideas also show up in Chapter 8, devoted to providing models of group treatments centered in exercises and techniques of positive psychology and focused on training to develop optimism and resilience. These approaches can be applied to both individual and group counseling.

## Helping Stuttering and TBI Children to Feel "Right" about Themselves

The following ten starting points, presented in no specific order of importance, are illustrative activities based on positive psychology exercises and adapted for use with Billy, a 10- to 12-year-old boy who stutters. All activities can be in written or spoken form, but of importance, they also must be discussed. Note that they do not address stuttering, and although not denying the stuttering at all, the counselor should discourage Billy from focusing the activities on it. They can be effectively used as topics for small-group discussions with Billy and other stutterers of similar age. These activities are suggested as adjuncts for more traditional therapies, not as substitutes for them. With appropriate adjustments, most are equally applicable to high-functioning children with TBI as well.

1. Give Billy the child version of the Values in Action measure (VIA) suggested in Chapter 2 (available at www.authentichap piness.org). Discuss the outcomes, and emphasize and exemplify the importance of knowing his strengths and of figuring out how to use them. Which ones is Billy sad about *not* having? What can he do about it? How can Billy use the strengths to leverage the not-so-strong points? Help Billy to understand the difference between not-strengths and weaknesses. Suggest that he use one of his signature strengths every day for a week, and report the results.

2. Find out who Billy's heroes are. What are their strengths? Why are they appealing? How can they become a metaphor? (Metaphor is a word for counselors, not Billy.) How can they be helpful to Billy in solving problems? For example, if Spider-Man were being bullied, what would he do? Or Captain Underpants, if he was facing these problems?[5]

3. Ask Billy to tell a story about his happiest day this year. What was so good about it? It didn't "just happen." What part did Billy play in making it so good?

---

[5]Dav Pilkey, who invented Captain Underpants, is a hero of mine. According to his website (www.pilkey.com), he grew up with LLD and later capitalized on his drawing skills to develop a loony and outrageous collection of childhood fantasy stories for kids that embody many principles of positive psychology.

4. Ask Billy to tell a story about something he did that made him very proud. What strengths did it show? Why is it good to be proud of oneself?

5. Ask Billy to tell three really good things about his parents, his siblings, or other people that he likes. When he goes home tonight, he is to thank his parents and siblings for them and report back.

6. If Billy has a bad day, help him to analyze why, looking out for the "thinking traps," mentioned in Chapter 2, with an extended analysis and application provided in Chapter 8). His bad days may be related largely to stuttering. When this is so, help him to remember that stuttering isn't the only thing. Don't focus on the stuttering—help him to dispute it and refute it.

7. Ask Billy to think of three good things that happened to him yesterday. How did he cause them to happen?

8. Talk to Billy about a person who has really been good to him. What did this person do? Have Billy figure out a short thank-you speech for this person, deliver it, and report back.

9. Ask Billy to choose a good friend, and list four reasons why he likes this person. Have Billy tell his friend.

10. What nice things does Ms. X (Billy's teacher) do? Billy's assignment is to thank her next time she does something nice, either for the class or for Billy himself.

These suggestions for simple but often highly effective interventions are based on understanding of communication disorders and their counseling, and on some awareness of developments in the field of positive psychology.

Specific counseling issues for children who stutter or who have had a TBI that can be addressed using a proactive approach. They include the following:

- *Self-advocacy.* Ylvisaker and Feeney (1998) urge the preparation of self-advocacy tapes, a practice in which Billy prepares a videotape that his teachers and other helping professionals can watch help them to understand him.
- *Handling teasing and bullying.* Teasing and bullying probably are universal burdens for those who are different, and young persons who stutter and especially those who have had a TBI seem to receive a disproportionate share. As a pos-

itivist, a counselor can help Billy to "toughen up," although not at the expense of failing to help him understand his teasers. For example, Billy can be supported to devise and practice three to five comebacks for teasers that could be useful to him—for example, "I bet you don't even know how to stutter! When you get as good as I am, we'll have a contest." Perhaps a lesson in walking away with dignity, or maybe a boxing lesson or weight training, would be useful. The handbook on childhood bullying by Yaruss, Murphy, Quesal, and Reardon (2004) is particularly helpful here. The clinician also can role-play with Billy, taking turns at bullying and receiving it.

■ *Setting tolerance levels for teasing: tattletale versus silent victim*. Malcolm Gladwell (2006) recently noted that one of childhood's most difficult lessons is learning the ins and outs of being a tattletale. This probably is particularly hard for children with disabilities as they deal with their insensitive peers. Have Billy work on how to handle telling on teasers and bullies: When is it right to tell the teacher? What level or amount of teasing demands it? What does not? What are the advantages and disadvantages of telling and not telling?

■ *Laughing lessons*. The healing power of laughter seems to be considerably underplayed in relationship to stuttering. Learning not only when but how to lighten up and how to help others to laugh are both skills that can be useful to stuttering children. Following are two examples:

a. Helping children to differentiate the big problems from the little ones, and the intermediate ones, is a proactive skill. To this end, create a series of mishap scenarios, some of which include stuttering. Have Billy evaluate the calamity factor of each, provide a solution, and determine if there is anything to laugh about in the mishap. An example follows:

You get mud on your new sneakers the very first time you wear them; you forget to defrost the hamburger like you promised your mother you'd do; you punch your sister when she calls you a dummy; the family cat knocked over a box of cereal, and because you were seen cleaning it up, your dad yells at you for spilling it.

Have Billy consult a joke book and find three jokes that he thinks are funny. Have him tell the jokes to five people, and evaluate their reactions.

■ *Education of peers and self-disclosure: speaking/writing about stuttering.* In cooperation with his teacher, work with Billy to prepare a short speech on stuttering to present to his class, or write a letter about stuttering to his classmates. The rationale for this activity is as follows: Helping Billy's classmates to understand his stuttering can help to allay any discomfort about it, thereby lessening the impetus for teasing. It also diverts focus from the stuttering person to his relatively minor flaw, and Billy's open acknowledgement and his appeal for support can undercut reasons for teasing. Billy should also be encouraged ask his classmates what they have learned from his presentation.

■ *Resilience training.* Approaches to resilience training for children have become available recently and are easily accessible by parents and by clinicians via www.reflective learning.org, as discussed in Chapters 2 and 8. Consider ways in which you can incorporate such training into the management of children with both early-onset and later-onset disorders.

## Conclusions

This chapter reviews the counseling needs of a wide range of families and children for whom onset of the communication disorder follows a period of normal language development. The use of stuttering and TBI as example disorders leaves readers to apply the information to a wider range of communication disorders in children, ranging from rare problems like Landau-Kleffner syndrome and other late-appearing hearing disorders to the more common ones such as SLI and phonological and voice disorders. It is crucial for the communication counselor to appreciate the distinction between disorders that are recognized at the time of birth in an infant at risk for communication disorders, or soon thereafter, and those that are recognized only later in life.

In keeping with my belief that the reader's creativity far exceeds mine, this approach and the counseling suggestions included here are not delineated completely, leaving the reader to move beyond the information presented and to enhance it with personal knowledge and experience.

## References

Bennett, E. (2006). *Working with people who stutter: A lifespan approach.* Upper Saddle River, NJ: Pearson Prentice Hall.

Bernstein Ratner, N., & Guitar, B. (2006). Treatment of very early stuttering and parent-administered therapy: The state of the art. In N. Bernstein Ratner & J. Tetnowski (Eds.), *Stuttering research and practice. Volume 2: Contemporary issues and approaches.* Mahwah, NJ: Lawrence Erlbaum.

Boss, P. (1999). *Ambiguous loss.* Cambridge, MA: Harvard.

Curlee, R. F., & Yairi, E. (1997). Early intervention with early childhood stuttering: A critical examination of the data. *American Journal of Speech-Language Pathology, 6,* 8–18.

Foundas, A. L., Bollich, A. M., Cory, D. M., Hurley, M., & Heilman, K. M. (2001). Anomalous anatomy of speech-language areas in adults with persistent developmental stuttering. *Neurology, 57,* 207–215.

Gladwell, M. (2006). Here's why: commentary on Charles Tilly's book Why? *New Yorker,* April 10.

Ingham, R. J., & Cordes, A. K. (1998). Treatment decisions for young children who stutter: Further concerns and complexities. *American Journal of Speech-Language Pathology, 7,* 10–19.

Jones, M., Onslow, M., Packman, A., Williams, S., Ormond, T., Schwarz, I., et al. (2005). Randomised controlled trial of the Lidcombe programme of early stuttering intervention. *British Medical Journal, 331,* 659–664.

Onslow, M. (2003). Evidence-based treatment of stuttering: IV. Empowerment through evidence-based treatment practices. *Journal of Fluency Disorders, 28,* 237–245.

Klein, E. & Amster, B. (2004). The effects of cognitive behavioral therapy with people who stutter. In A. Packman, A. Meltzer, & H. Peters (Eds.), *Theory, research and fluency disorders: The fourth world congress of fluency disorders* (p. 154–160). Nijmegen Netherlands: Nijmegen Press.

Onslow, M., & Packman, A. (1999). (Eds.). *The handbook of early stuttering intervention.* San Diego, CA: Singular Publishing Group.

Onslow, M., Packman, A. & Harrison, E. (2003). *The Lidcombe Program of early stuttering intervention: A clinician's guide.* Austin, TX: Pro-Ed.

Ratner, N. (2005). Evidence based practice in stuttering: Some questions to consider. *Journal of Fluency Disorders, 30,* 164–188.

Rogers, F. (2003). *The world according to Mister Rogers: Important things to remember.* New York: Hyperion.

Seligman, M. E. P. (2002). *Authentic happiness.* New York: Free Press.

Sheehan, J. G. (1970). *Stuttering: Research and therapy.* New York: Harper & Row.

Sommer, M., Koch, M. A., Paulus, W., Weiller, C., & Buchel, C. (2002). Disconnection of speech-relevant brain areas in persistent developmental stuttering. *Lancet, 360,* 380–386.

Yaruss, S., Murphy, B., Quesal, R., & Reardon, N. (2004). *Bullying and teasing: Helping children who stutter.* New York: National Stuttering Association.

Ylvisaker, M., & Feeney, T. (1998). *Collaborative brain injury intervention: Positive everyday routines.* San Diego, CA: Singular Publishing Group.

## Websites

www.biausa.org

www.friendswhostutter.org

www.nsastutter.org

www.neuro.pmr.vcu.edu

www.pilkey.com

www.russhicks.com

www.stutteringhomepage.com

www.talkinghelp.org

www3.fhs.usyd.edu.au/asrcwww/treatment/lidcombe.htm

## *Chapter 6*

# COMMUNICATION COUNSELING WITH ADULT CLIENTS AND THEIR FAMILIES FOR WHOM PROGRESSION IS TOWARD IMPROVEMENT

*E*xcept for perhaps stuttering treated in adulthood and some adult-onset voice disorders, most adult communication disorders result from specific medical conditions. A close look at adult problems from a holistic perspective reveals two general patterns of progression that have profound implications for counseling: improvement (indicated by physical or functional recovery or stabilization, or both) and deterioration.

With disorders characterized by the first pattern, affected persons have a high probability of getting better, if only somewhat, with the passage of time. With certain more or less obvious exceptions, such as metastatic brain cancer, the prognosis is never worse than when it is initially incurred. In conditions that result from brain damage involving cerebrovascular disease, the excision of a nonmalignant brain tumor, or the consequences of traumatic brain injury (TBI), a change toward the better may be termed "spontaneous recovery," which reflects neuroplasticity. For clients whose communication or swallowing disorder is secondary to conditions such as laryngectomy, a more appropriate term may be "healing." All of these conditions probably involve new learning and adaptation over time as well. Counseling clients with disorders that fit this more positive pattern is explored in this chapter.

Disorders characterized by the second pattern of deterioration have an inevitably downward progression or may be fatal. Affected persons have a high likelihood of getting worse to some degree with the passage of time, despite appropriate treatment and intervention. Such disorders are the focus of Chapter 7.

An advantage of counseling adults with disorders of upward progression over counseling parents and children with communication disorders is that from the start, outcomes seem a bit more clear, even though similar crises are initially evident. Furthermore, most adult disorders occur in midlife or thereafter, thereby constraining lifespan considerations. This is not meant to minimize the counseling concerns for persons whose problems occur later in life and have a somewhat more predictable course. Rather, it simply underscores the reality that these disorders have different counseling priorities. Issues such as the likelihood of returning to work, altered family roles, retirement, social isolation, and lifestyle restrictions and changes now arise, in part supplanting more general issues such as safety, acceptance, and fulfillment, as discussed in Chapter 4.

Age also differentiates parent/child counseling in communication disorders from counseling with adults. Rather than working with children, and perhaps counseling parents who are likely to be from the clinician's own generation, now clinicians may be counseling adults nearer to the age of their parents or grandparents. Generational differences between counselors and clients do not necessarily present problems, but they may be dicey, particularly when counselors are younger than those whom they counsel. Counseling responsibilities to adults with these disorders also extend to older spouses and partners and possibly, grown children. For younger counselors, especially, it is essential to keep in mind that good counseling with older adults grows from a foundation of healthy respect for one's elders and knowledge about the aging process.

This chapter highlights adult communication disorders that occur following stroke. It emphasizes aphasia, apraxia of speech, right hemisphere cognitive-communication disorders, dysphagia, and dysarthria. Stroke is the focus because it is the most common cause of this pattern of communication disorders. However, the counseling approach should be equally applicable to adults with TBIs, speech disorders resulting from cancer of the larynx and other adult communication disorders in which improvement over the passage of time can be comfortably assumed.

Because this chapter concerns the multiple consequences of a single type of event, it starts with a brief discussion of specific stroke features that affect communication counseling. Next it discusses communication problems that follow stroke. The varying counseling needs of persons who experience stroke and their caregivers are then related to the time course of recovery. Aphasia serves as the focus disorder.

## Stroke and Communication Counseling

What aspects of stroke in and of itself are important to communication counseling? Some issues are in the background but are likely to influence the tone of communication counseling covertly, but pervasively. Others are questions to which counselors need to provide answers.

### Background Issues

Two broad concerns lurk in the background: First, stroke has seriously threatened the affected person's life, with implications for both that person and the spouse or family; and second, stroke changes priorities, sometimes unavoidably. Each is discussed next.

■ *Stroke is a brush with death, and a reminder of the transience of life, for both the person who experiences stroke and the family.*

Even the term "stroke survivor" reflects the drastic nature of the event. For most people, such events—stroke, serious head injury, or detection of cancer, for example—are bound up with issues of death and dying and may serve as wake-up calls to live more fully and more wholesomely, or may lead to reaffirmation of religious faith. A stroke is frightening for persons who experience one, as well as for people around them. Fear and anxiety center on the apprehension that another stroke will occur; such feelings often are the culprits in instances of overprotection and disproportionate cautiousness. Capable communication counselors must acknowledge fear and anxiety but be prepared to supply antidotes, ranging from providing useful simple information to helping affected persons engage in activities designed to reduce their distress. Chapter 8 includes such an activity, centered on the familiar concern of family members' fear of leaving their aphasic family member alone. The activity uses a model called "real-time resilience" by Reivich and Shatté (2002). It is an extremely useful approach in the group workshop format described in Chapter 8 but it is also useful for individual counseling.

■ *Stroke changes reality.*

Communication disorders, as well as many of stroke's other accompaniments, result in major lifestyle changes for many people. These include new worries about finances, role changes, living arrangements, social life, leisure time, driving, and many more. At least some such factors exist for every stroke family, and each of them underscores the need for helping families to develop resilience and optimism, and to reestablish a sense of self.

## Foreground Issues

In addition to background issues, there are usually two major immediate concerns for affected persons and their families. Neither the causes nor the effects of stroke generally are well known to most people. Both influence recovery and require explication. Each is discussed next from a counseling perspective.

■ *What is a stroke, anyway?*

As noted in Chapter 1, this question seems particularly pertinent early in the recovery process. The crisis atmosphere immediately surrounding stroke often makes it difficult for patients and families to absorb even simple and accurate explanations, because they are experiencing shock. Of interest, even when the information has apparently gotten through, affected persons and families for whom the stroke is in the distant past seldom are bored by the topic and continue to listen intently as the information is presented again, for example, in spouse groups. Both hearing the general stroke facts repetitively and reiterating one's own stroke story appear to reduce fear and anxiety. Telling the story again and again also seems to emphasize the distance traveled on the road to successful management, and revisiting the topic is reassuring. Revisits to stroke facts always should include information about latest treatments. See Box 6.1.

■ *Why did it happen to me? to us?*

Of relevance here, the preferred term today is *stroke*, rather than "cerebrovascular accident (CVA)," according to the American Stroke Association (ASA), an affiliate of the American Heart Association, as well as the National Stroke Association (NSA). Both agencies object

---

**Box 6.1 Guidelines for Telling the Stroke Story**

1. Write a new story.
   a. Eliminate professional jargon.
   b. Use diagrams.
   c. Include risk factors and warning signs and what to do about them.
   d. Goal is empowerment, not threat.
2. Practice your new story with your family or some friends.
   a. Tell it simply and clearly.
   b. Seek confirmation about what they understood.
   c. Get their feedback.
   d. Provide written materials to accompany your stroke story.

to the notion of "accident," emphasizing instead that stroke has known risk factors, and that prevention of stroke involves being aware of risk factors and engaging in wellness behaviors that mitigate them. Alertness to signs that a stroke is impending also is stressed. In fact, the NSA lobbies for the term *brain attack*, equating it with "heart attack," to underscore the urgency of recognizing early stroke symptoms and getting help immediately.

Programs aimed at prevention are of undeniable importance. Communication counselors, however, are involved with people who have *not* prevented stroke. These clients need to understand how and why it happened, perhaps to prevent a recurrence but perhaps also to deal with blame and guilt. How did it happen? Modifiable risk factors may have not been recognized. Or perhaps the person who had the stroke did not follow physician recommendations to make lifestyle changes, or perhaps the spouse or other family members also were unaware of risks, or failed to make them clear or to support needed changes. Perhaps risk factors were attended to and the stroke happened anyway.

In any case, guilt and anger may rule. In fact, guilt and anger often compete, and often depression raises its ugly post-stroke head as well. A personal story illustrates these dynamics:

> My former husband, a neurologist and far more knowledgeable about stroke than I, suffered a stroke. As an experienced aphasiologist, I was well aware of risk factors, and I knew (as did he) that being overweight, lack of exercise, eating a questionable diet and drinking excessively were problematical. All were in play, and I was worried.
>
> Did I point all this out? Of course. Did I make a convincing case? No. I tried, unsuccessfully, or at least not in time. Was my failure to convince him due to the possibility he was rejecting what I had to say because I was a nag? Possibly. Was it due to the fact that I made my case poorly? Also possibly.
>
> After the stroke, how did he feel? Guilty because he knew better, for sure. And embarrassed—this should not have happened to a knowledgeable neurologist. But in relation to a few risk factors (not all), he subsequently changed his ways. Finally, he was angry with me for being right (as well as unsuccessful in suppressing "I told you so"). And he was depressed, a natural consequence of stroke.

After the stroke, where was I emotionally? I was scared. I was angry because he had not listened to me. I felt guilty because I had not made my case appropriately. I felt totally powerless. Despite the fact that my husband returned to work, did the stroke influence our relationship? You bet.

His stroke had relatively minimal physical and functional consequences, none of which involved communication. Nevertheless, those questions lingered, unanswered and unresolved, for a long time into our healing process.

My story is merely a vehicle for pointing out that a complex dynamic is likely to underlie the apparently simple question of "Why did this happen to me?" The complexity has substantial potential to influence not only counseling but the course of intervention as well.

## Accompanying Problems

It is well known that in addition to the communication problems that result from stroke, physical and cognitive effects also can complicate the counseling picture. This section summarizes some ways in which these effects interact with our counseling responsibilities.

### Mobility

Because of their focus on communication, SLP-As sometimes are rather dismissive of the burdens imposed by paralysis on stroke persons and families. Mobility issues may serve as strong deterrents to receiving outpatient care and often contribute to family fatigue. And hard as it may be for some of us in this profession to believe, mobility problems may be more important than communication problems for some people who have had a stroke For example, an aphasic man from our aphasia clinic who before his stroke was an avid hunter and fisherman took his aphasia in stride—but he was devastated by his inability to pursue the outdoor life. Possibly the best thing that happened in his aphasia rehabilitation was when he and his clinician jointly researched, found, and evaluated adaptive fishing rods and handicapped-accessible fishing piers. He also provides a good example of how to intertwine counseling and direct language work.

## Cognition

Cognitive problems that sometimes accompany stroke may be elusive in some cases and confounding in others. The slogan of the Adler Aphasia Center, located in Maywood, New Jersey, is "Aphasia: Loss of words, not intellect." This wording reflects a point of view that is well engrained in SLPs, for the good reason that in most cases it is true. When a person has incurred many strokes, however, or when stroke occurs in a person who has had previous cognitive decline, this picture may be altered. Furthermore, persons with severe global aphasia, complicated possibly by dysarthria and apraxia of speech, also have increased probability of the co-occurrence of additional neuropsychological problems such as difficulty in problem solving (Helm-Estabrooks, 2002). Moreover, in such persons, because of the extent of their language deficits, additional problems may be particularly difficult to identify and to treat.

Clients with right hemisphere brain damage (RHD) also present significant challenges in this regard. First, they share the characteristics of disorganized, egocentric, pragmatically compromised, tangential, and digressive language use with dementing persons and those with TBI. "Cognitive communication disorders" is our shorthand for implying that their language has links to more extensive (if sometimes subtle) impairments. And of course, impairments such as anosognosia and neglect of the left hemi space complicate the cognitive picture for RHD people as well.[1]

Denial and anosognosia in persons with RHD require special consideration. The question "When is a problem a problem?" can occur across the spectrum of adult communication disorders, but

---

[1]The most extensive interaction among language and cognitive problems of course occurs with TBI, as pointed out in Chapter 5, and with dementias, described in Chapter 7. Very few adults who have incurred TBI develop frank aphasia; even fewer persons with dementia do. To the contrary, in most cases, the psychosocial consequences of the disorders are simply made manifest through language and language problems.

it is especially urgent in RHD and possibly in TBI as well. Many cognitive-communicative manifestations of RHD may be subtle and minimally apparent to casual acquaintances. Clearly, their presence is a counseling concern, and there are ethical considerations as well. No general answer is possible here, but how a "problem" is defined and who defines it as such constitute important issues for communication counselors.

## Psychiatric/Psychological Issues

According to the National Institute of Mental Health (2006), depression is estimated to have a prevalence of between 10% and 27%, increasing by 15% to 40% in the first two months after stroke. Depression therefore is a major concern, because when it occurs, it can impede the rehabilitation process. If depression is suspected, clinicians must bring it to the immediate attention of physicians, who may prescribe antidepressant medication. Two such drugs have been shown to be particularly effective with stroke. tricyclic antidepressants (TCAs) and selective serotonin reuptake inhibitors (SSRIs).

Although "talking therapies" have a respected role in the management of depression in general, they are of limited use in persons with stroke-related language and speech disorders. In some instances, co-treatment conducted by a mental health specialist and an SLP can be beneficial, but this is a luxury for most. The most important consideration for communications counselors regarding post-stroke depression is to be alert for its signs in both affected persons *and* family members and to refer appropriately if it is found. It also is essential to provide a supportive environment for post-stroke clients and their families who are experiencing depression as they participate in treatment for communication disorders. The three possible sources for depression after stroke are listed in Box 6.2.

## Psychosocial Issues

Box 6.2 makes it clear that people can be depressed before a stroke or can incur depression as a consequence. Other factors also can

---

**Box 6.2 Sources of Depression in Stroke**

■ Depression can occur as a neural accompaniment of stroke.
■ Depression can occur as a reaction to stroke.*
■ Depression can precede the stroke.*

---

*In family members too, of course.

---

be involved as well. For example, strokes can happen to people with bad marriages, nasty personalities, and decidedly unhelpful children. Stroke has seldom been known to solve such problems or to alter such circumstances favorably. Rather, they become counseling issues.

Although it is not an inevitable consequence, social isolation frequently affects people who have had a stroke, particularly those with resultant aphasia. Along with other consequences of aging, the slipping away of friends and social contacts is also a particularly cruel aftermath of stroke. One of the most beneficial results of participation in stroke and aphasia groups (and spouse groups as well) is that it breaks this chain of loneliness. In many instances, deep friendships are formed and extend beyond the contacts made in groups.

A review of risk factors for stroke is appropriate here: advancing age, high blood pressure, tobacco use, diabetes, carotid artery disease, sickle cell disease, high blood levels of "bad" cholesterol and low levels of "good" cholesterol, obesity, physical inactivity, excessive alcohol intake, and drug use. This list of risk factors supports the notion that stroke is hardly an equal opportunity disease. The relative prevalence rates for differing socioeconomic levels in the United States make it clear that stroke does not statistically favor America's "rich and famous." Statistical trends do not predict individual patterns and variability, but this list of risk factors suggests that many economic and social problems can accompany stroke and influence its counseling.

In the following case example, the affected person does *not* fit a predictable stroke pattern, but some of the possible counseling concerns are well illustrated:

> Matt Z is an upper-middle-class, 65-year-old white man who did not smoke and who worked out regularly, ate very carefully, drank moderately, and had unremarkable findings on yearly

physical examinations. He held a powerful position in a major company and was reputed to have had fairly contentious relationships with his colleagues and subordinates. Following his retirement, Mr. Z and his wife, Clara, moved to Arizona, where he began to indulge his passion, golf. Six months later, he had a moderately severe right hemisphere stroke, with resulting significant cognitive and communicative consequences and severe left hemiplegia.

Clara Z, his now bewildered and vaguely angry wife, is 15 years his junior and came to Arizona with him to play golf and to enjoy the rich social life available in their community. Mr. Z's three children from a previous marriage are somewhat concerned about him but do not seem to grasp the details of his situation, and they all live far away; moreover, their relationship with him is rather strained because they are still confused about why he divorced their mother 10 years earlier.

As an exercise, examine the psychosocial features that could influence Mr. Z's recovery, even in the absence of a detailed clinical assessment of his RHD. Determine those that play a role in counseling both husband and wife. Successful communication counselors should try to be aware of all of the factors that influence successful treatment and recovery, and to be prepared to deal with them.

This rapid sweep through the broad territory of stroke should alert clinicians to the idea that although a specific person's speech and language profile affects the post-stroke clinical course, interventions, counseling, and outcome, there are many other influences as well. Indeed, most medical problems occur in complex contexts, such as with TBI, cancer, and kidney disease. Such complexity reminds us that our goals are to treat people, not their impairments.

## Communication Problems after Stroke

This book is biased toward communication problems. This chapter is particularly biased in its insistence that communication disorders are stroke's most devastating consequence. But outside of our own profession, communication problems are likely to be stroke's most easily marginalized consequences. Why is this so?

Communication, like breathing, is pervasive and frequently is taken for granted. As a result, even most health care professionals fail to recognize the extent to which communication problems can have profound negative effects on quality of life. Sadly, this remains true for most people until communication problems personally affect them. Families also take communication for granted and fail to recognize the potentially catastrophic effects of communication problems before they experience them.

The marginalization ceases with a stroke that results in communication problems. For most people, talking and thinking are practically synonymous. Loss of ability to talk well may be construed as an indication that thinking also is compromised. Furthermore, one's identity and sense of self are muted or altered when the means to express them are limited—hence the sage advice of the Adler Center motto.

The foregoing reflects the darker side of the stroke experience. But there is also a lighter side. Stroke is an example of the Zorba-like notion of the "full catastrophe." As borne out my own clinical experience, the negative effect on the lives of aphasic persons and their families often can be tempered or neutralized by behaviors concerning some particular "stroke fact" thought to be otherwise immutable. What particular people bring to stroke and to other potentially devastating conditions is as important as what the disorders bring.

Additional support for this perspective comes from stories from other professionals and reports written by stroke persons and their families, along with websites relating to their recovery. Brief stories of persons who have brought personal strengths and unique attitudes to their recovery include the following: Roger Ross (2007) essentially neutralized his aphasia by devoting himself to developing aphasia groups for others to attend. Mike and Elaine Adler put their energies to work to build the Adler Aphasia Center after Mike's stroke (www.adleraphasiacenter.org). Eileen Quann chronicled her experiences as a spouse in a way that extends her helpful hand to other stroke families (2002). Tommye Mayer (2000) and Paul Berger with Stephanie Mensch (1999) each wrote a very helpful and practical book about living with hemiplegia. Robert McCrum chronicled his right-hemisphere stroke (1999). Kirk Douglas described getting on with his life as a person with dysarthria (2003). One amazing final example is that of Dorothea Wender, a professor of classics who had an aphasia-producing stroke. Dr. Wender wrote inspiring stories of her recovery and published her own experiment on the efficacy of her self-designed and self-delivered therapy in a major neurology journal (1989).

Not all people greet stroke or its aftermath as challenges, nor are they constitutional optimists, nor do they do heroic things or write books about their stroke experiences. Many are simply every-day folks who live successfully with aphasia, learning to take life's setbacks in stride and serving as role models for their peers. (A number of such stroke stories can be found in the journal *Topics in Stroke Rehabilitation*, volume 13.1, 2006.) Of particular note is the extensive group of personal stories available in the literature that were collected by Hinckley (2006). Box 6.3 describes one of the most moving experiences I have experienced in this regard.

The good news is that counseling, coaching, and strong peer support all can help those who are overwhelmed, helpless and hopeless. People can be aided to see things differently, to capitalize on their strengths, and to develop some degree of resilience as a result. This is the bright side of counseling, but one not often rec-ognized or emphasized.

## Counseling for Aphasia, Right Hemisphere Cognitive Disorders, Dysarthria, and Apraxia of Speech: Differing Goals at Different Times

As persons with communication disorders begin their journey toward some degree of resolution, they and their clinicians both need to be reminded once again that no one knows how far along that path anyone may travel. In counseling post-stroke clients, the crystal ball is always cloudy. Not only is it unethical to pretend otherwise, but facilitating false hope also is cruel. Nevertheless, because the post-stroke clinical course progresses positively over time, some substantial recovery from aphasia, RHD, apraxia of speech, dysphagia, and dysarthria can be expected. This is particu-larly likely to occur with appropriate intervention (see Robey, 1998, for information on efficacy of aphasia rehabilitation, for example). Families and individuals with communication disorders must be made explicitly aware of positive change and encouraged to watch for it—not full recovery necessarily, but changes in that direction. Progression toward improvement also implies that change

**Box 6.3**
**Everyday Resilience: Clinical Example**

A large group of aphasic individuals and their families had assembled for a Workshop on aphasia. I was the group leader, and I knew nobody in the room except a clinician or two, and most of the families were strangers to each other as well. I began by introducing myself and telling a bit of my story, and then I suggested we go around the room and share stories with each other. My job was simply to highlight important stroke facts, or aphasia truisms that the stories were revealing, particularly those that were likely to have meaning for others in the room. Not surprisingly, some people found it easy to talk; others were more reticent. Sometimes it was the person with aphasia who spoke, sometimes the spouse or caregiver, and sometimes both, and as we went along, the discussion warmed with shared experiences.

Finally, it was the turn of a man whose aphasia had almost totally resolved, and he told his story, starting with the previous day, day when he retook his real estate examination and began the process of returning to work. Then he said: "But now I want to tell you something really important. I have had two events in my life that I viewed as personal disasters. The first was when I was drafted to fight in Vietnam, and the second was when I had my stroke two years ago. As I look back now, I realize that they were the most important events in my life. I hated both of them. They were both awful, but they were what I have learned the most from. They taught me what is life is about and why I should cherish it. And they taught me who I am."

There was silence. I was too close to tears to attempt to break it. Then a woman who had already talked, and had told us that she was talking for her husband George as well as for herself because he could not talk at all, said: "All I can say is thank you. I never told you this before, George, but your stroke is the most important thing that has happened to me, too. It taught me what love is."

itself may result in differing counseling agendas at different times. Counselors must be prepared to accommodate change. Accordingly, counseling issues for three time intervals are discussed next: first at the onset of aphasia, during the acute phase; then during its rehabilitation phase; and finally, during its chronic phase. These phases and changing agendas are relevant to aphasia, dysarthria, and apraxia of speech, but for simplicity, aphasia is used here as an exemplar.

With RHD, timing of counseling to issues as they arise is not quite so simple. Specifically, unless the stroke and its consequences leave severe right hemisphere impairments such as extensive anosognosia or hemispatial neglect, many of its communication consequences may be somewhat masked at the onset and become a concern only during rehabilitation or in chronic phases. Nevertheless, if the problems experienced early on by the client with RHD are relevant, then the counseling principles presented next are appropriate.

## Counseling at the Onset

A series of questions appropriate for these three time periods was recently developed (Avent, Glista, Wallace, Jackson, Nishioka, & Yip, 2005) and their utility subsequently was evaluated (Avent, Glista, Wallace, & Johnson, submitted for publication). The questions initially were identified in work with focus groups of families, and in the evaluation study, additional families, along with persons uninformed about stroke and aphasia and SLPs judged the relative importance of each of the questions isolated in the development study. (As discussed later, as they also looked at questions that arise on discharge from formal rehabilitation work.) The onset-phase questions judged by 90% of the families to be extremely important are presented in Box 6.4.

In effect, this list constitutes the informational agenda for communication counselors who work with stroke families. Certainly, answers should be provided, in many forms using various media, as noted in Chapter 1 and earlier in this chapter.[2]

---

[2]How do *you* explain aphasia to your patients and families? It is even more foreign than stroke, and murkier to explain, as just suggested. Practice your answers. Write them. Hand them out.

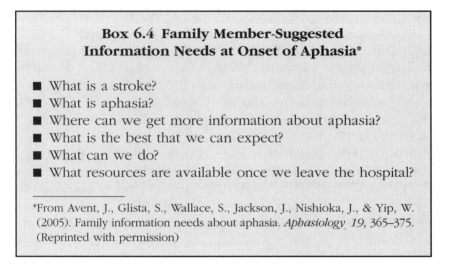

**Box 6.4 Family Member-Suggested Information Needs at Onset of Aphasia***

- What is a stroke?
- What is aphasia?
- Where can we get more information about aphasia?
- What is the best that we can expect?
- What can we do?
- What resources are available once we leave the hospital?

*From Avent, J., Glista, S., Wallace, S., Jackson, J., Nishioka, J., & Yip, W. (2005). Family information needs about aphasia. *Aphasiology, 19*, 365–375. (Reprinted with permission)

Nevertheless, the Box 6.4 questions are retrospective; that is, study participants are looking back on their remembered informational needs, not on what they were actively seeking during the earliest days of the experience. In fact, the complex psychodynamics of the early grief period probably preclude clear memories. Taking advantage of information in the early phases of crisis probably is not possible for most families. Therefore, simply providing answers those questions is not enough. Information should be supplemented by two of the other counseling activities presented in Chapter 1: receiving information that the affected person and family wish to share, and helping them to clarify their ideas and feelings. The fourth activity, providing options for changing behaviors, is premature at the onset of stroke, in fact, a particularly delicate counseling task is to help people understand why detailed planning probably should wait, at least for a bit. Relevant counseling activities also include simply listening to concerns about the future, sharing sadness and frustration, offering the immediate help that the clinician feels is within the scope of practice for counseling, being supportive, and holding the client's hand.

## Acute Intervention: Getting off to a Good Start

Julius Fridriksson and I have written extensively (and controversially[3]) about early treatment after onset of aphasia (Holland &

[3]See a rebuttal to this article by Peach (2001).

Fridricksson, 2001). Put briefly, our contention is that in the acute phase of stroke, clinicians should intersperse and intertwine counseling as described above, with direct intervention. That is, communication counselors should use clinical encounters to get patients and families off to a good start. We urge the use of activities that can illustrate spontaneous recovery to patients and families, and that are embedded into the familiar medium of conversation, to emphasize what the affected person can still do in the earliest days following stroke, despite aphasia. These principles are briefly described next.

### *Illustrating Spontaneous Recovery*

Families and patients (they are still "patients" at this point in their recovery) are not well positioned to understand the language behaviors that comprise communication impairments. Talking about spontaneous recovery and change probably won't get through. *Showing* families and patients what is happening, rather than just *telling* them about it, is likely to be more effective. It is possible to illustrate for families and patients what spontaneous recovery is all about, focusing on aspects of communication that are still intact, rather than on what language is currently not retrievable.

How can we illustrate spontaneous recovery? One way is by taking note of daily changes (preferably using repetitive activities) and bringing the changes to the attention of both aphasic persons and their families. For example, the clinician may state:

> "Mr. Jones, that was great! Mrs. Jones, yesterday when I saw your husband, I asked him what your name was, and I didn't understand what he said. And today, when you walked in, he said 'Hi, Maude' clear as a bell. Did you both notice that? Mr. Jones, give yourself a pat on the back for the progress! Changes like that even have a name—'spontaneous recovery' (*write it*). Glad to see it's kicking in."

Rather than practicing abstract drills and such, using repetitive activities incorporated into conversation can reveal small daily changes. The goal is to capitalize on communication strengths, rather than to lay bare communication impairments.

### Using Conversation

The reason for embedding such tasks into conversation is that conversation is natural. Even in the earliest days after stroke, conversation encourages even marginal strengths to emerge. By focusing on this natural process, clinicians can help aphasic persons and their families to mitigate the "identity theft"—Shadden's term (2005)—that results when adults develop communication disorders. Shadden also notes that although clinicians always believe they support their client's sense of competency, "we use labels that point to incompetence, and recognize our clients for their impairment" (p. 219). Our clinical tasks often also highlight impairment. Therefore, particularly in the very early phases after stroke, it is crucial to highlight what is *right*, rather than what is wrong. Clinicians should focus on preserved behaviors, and do it in the most naturalistic way, by encouraging talking and conversation.

### Activities for Acute Treatment

The foregoing has been a brief summary of an approach detailed by Holland and Fridriksson (2001). Many additional suggestions for activities are provided there. Box 6.5 samples some that are consistent with this approach to early management. Some of the activities are designed to involve families, and thus aimed at answering the question raised by Avent and colleagues (2005) about what families can do to help. Others are suggestions for clinicians.

### Documenting and Data

It is important to keep careful track of daily changes and improvements. They become part of the progress notes, but they also should be shared with families, patients, and other staff members. Such documentation is the written record of spontaneous recovery and of behavioral strengths.

Holland & Fridriksson (2001) formalized the approach just described and collected some data to support its effectiveness when acute care stays lasted longer than a week.[4] There is now considerably more urgency concerning how to provide counseling

---

[4]And that was not during World War I—it was about 1990!

### Box 6.5 Suggested Activities for Post-Stroke Clients and Families*

The case of Mrs. M, who suffered a stroke two days previously and has aphasia, is used as an example.

**Activities for family members:**

- Explain that keeping track of what Mrs. M says, and how well she seems to understand, would be very useful. Provide a small notebook and a pencil, and ask family members to record what was said, when, and a very brief summary of the circumstances. Give examples, and ask them to leave the notebook in the room for your use when you come in each day. Also, use the notebook to communicate with them.
- Ask family to write a brief "story" of Mrs. M—her work and interests, some things about the family and other significant people, family member names, some likes and pet peeves, TV habits, and so on.

**Activities for clients/acute care clinicians:**

- *Comprehension*: Fill in the menu form together; ask Mrs. M some relevant questions that you know the answers to (perhaps from the brief story above); provide sequential commands involving objects in the room. Use Mrs. M's responses as the basis for charting. Provide feedback concerning appropriateness and differences from previous day.
- *Reading*: Read get-well cards, daily schedules, or menus together; check for amount of support required. As with comprehension activities, keep track of Mrs. M's responses for her chart, and provide feedback.
- *Spoken language*: Check family names; watch some TV together and ask questions about what is happening; hold relevant simple conversations. As for other components of monitoring, track Mrs. M's responses and provide feedback.
- *Speech production*: Note changes in dysarthria or apraxia of speech in Mrs. M's speech; track and provide feedback.

■ *Swallowing*—the centerpiece of acute care: If the clinician is feeding or observing Mrs. M during meals, it is the best time to practice conversation as well (between careful chewing, chin tucks, and other self-protection maneuvers), and also check on comprehension.

*Modified slightly from Holland, A., & Fridriksson, J. (2001). Management for aphasia in the acute phases post stroke. *American Journal of Speech-Language Pathology, 10*(1), 19-28.

in the constrained time frame that characterizes present lengths of hospital stay. One goal is answering the important questions, but the other is getting off to a good start. To enter a rehabilitation center with a little of one's self-esteem and self-efficacy intact is a tremendous boost to recovery.

## Moving to Rehabilitation

People should now lose their "patient" (i.e., helpless) designation. Health care professionals appear to expect that people will improve significantly if they work hard enough in rehabilitation. SLPs now abet the "good start" with the "power of therapy." Another subtle message comes along with this one: that rehabilitation is where the recovery action is. This is partially true, but to maximize it, and to prepare for the future, there are two early tasks for communication counselors. One task concerns the expectations of affected persons and their families about rehabilitation: "dispelling rehabilitation magic." The other task concerns learning the rehabilitation ropes: "solving the rehabilitation mystery." In what follows, counseling involves not only a set of tools but also a specific attitude. This is not an accident; it feels contextually appropriate to the fast pace of rehabilitation. ("Counseling moments" haven't been abandoned; they are picked up by the boxful later in this chapter.)

### *Expectations: Dispelling Rehabilitation Magic*

At the onset of aphasia (see Box 6.4), families have already asked, "What is the best we can expect?" (Avent et al., 2005). This question still looms large at the beginning of speech and language treatment. Not only is the question scary for families and people with aphasia, but it also constitutes a challenge for clinicians because it puts them on the tightrope between offering false hope and projecting Eeyore-type gloom and doom. The question requires an answer. It demands forthrightness about saying "I don't know" while simultaneously acknowledging the importance of hope and the need to be optimistic.

Most rehabilitationists convey the notion that rehabilitation is a kind of endgame—that is, when rehabilitation is over, that is the end of positive change. At least that is what many families and persons with chronic aphasia report their beliefs to have been. This begins to explain their frustration and despair when formal rehabilitation ends and aphasia still lingers.

Certainly the structure of health care reimbursement plays a huge role in this misperception. Clinicians must stay attuned to the energy of the disability movement, the shared expertise, and the outburst of activity concerning chronic aphasia and then pass the word along to clients. They are key players in developing the optimism that permits families and aphasic people to grow and change after rehabilitation ends.

Rehabilitation is but the first significant step on the long road to living successfully after stroke. It is critical to communicate that message to the people with whom we work. Rehabilitation is not the final step in recovery. It is not wholly where recovery action is. It is not magic. Clinicians must convey the message that life indeed goes on after rehabilitation, and in most cases, life can continue to get better, particularly if attention is paid to aphasia in its chronic stages. When clients and families are encouraged not to expect magic, they are far less likely to be disappointed and discouraged.

### Solving the Rehabilitation Mystery: Learning the Rehabilitation Ropes

Just as rehabilitation is not magic, it should not be a mystery either. Box 6.6 lists family members' needs at the outset of speech-language treatment—that is, when clients enter rehabilitation.

At this point, families and aphasic clients are still new not only to aphasia but to the routines and goals of rehabilitation. My clinical experience indicates that a majority do not fully understand what the therapy process entails. Accordingly, clinicians need to explain why tests are given, and also what the treatment is expected to

**Box 6.6 Family Member-Suggested Information Needs at Onset of Speech-Language Treatment***

- What is the purpose of testing?
- What is the purpose of treatment?
- Can we watch or participate in therapy?
- How can we improve interactions?
- How can we help?
- What other things should we be aware of?
- Is there someone we can talk to who has gone through this?

*From Avent, J., Glista, S., Wallace, S., Jackson, J., Nishioka, J., & Yip, W. (2005). Family information needs about aphasia. *Aphasiology, 19*, 365–375.

accomplish.[5] Communication counselors need to view families and aphasic persons as fellow experts who can be extremely informative during treatment. Shadden points out that counselors need to know something about "the relational dynamics in families, going well beyond questions such as 'How does he communicate at home?'"(2005). Issues such as this all require counseling skills.

Families need instruction in *supported communication* (Kagan, 1998) during formal rehabilitation. In my experience, this typically is postponed until aphasia has become chronic—and thus *after* the affected person's sense of self has been damaged (although it could have been protected by this approach) (Holland & Beeson, 1993). Is there peer support for families undergoing rehabilitation, or will it have to wait until after rehabilitation? How do we help families to find information and peer support? These are counseling tasks as well.

Rehabilitation is better and easier to tolerate when the participants clearly understand it and consider themselves part of the process. The list of family needs in Box 6.6 also underscores families' concerns about what they should to be doing in the baffling new situation called rehabilitation. For aphasic persons in a rehabilitation center, the daily routine entails living in rooms with strangers;

---

[5]In many instances, the explanations we give to others also can clarify our own understanding of why we do what we do.

following a relatively rigid schedule; wearing clothes that are possibly unacceptable in one's everyday sartorial world; sitting across a table from a clinician likely to be the age of one's child (or grandchild); and following directions to participate in drills and school-like tasks; not being able to lie down and rest when tired; and eating from a limited menu. The rehabilitation milieu can certainly be managed more comfortably if its participants understand its rules, its goals, and its processes. (And language disorders probably complicate every aspect of this understanding.)

Furthermore, family members and aphasic persons themselves know very little about aphasia before it happens to them, even if Uncle Ted had a stroke some years ago and had trouble talking. One reason for this lack of knowledge is that *aphasia* is scarcely a household word (neither are *cognitive-communication problem*, *dysphagia*, *apraxia of speech*, or *dysarthria*, for that matter). Furthermore, the sense of crisis may be overwhelming, and the cause of the aphasia, unlike a natural disaster or even a well-publicized illness with glamorous spokespersons such as breast cancer, hardly makes it exotic. Finally, because of aphasia's variability, Uncle Ted's problems probably will not be particularly relevant.[6]

Particularly if they buy into "rehabilitation magic" and are bewildered by "rehabilitation mystery," both aphasic persons and their family members may very well feel uninformed and confused. In such instances, clinical intervention is not likely to be very meaningful, follow-through is negligible, and effectiveness is minimized. Such situations constitute is fertile ground for "counseling moments" to occur, and such encounters should be encouraged. If therapy just "happens," without both family and patient buy-in, clinical effectiveness is minimized. Consider the following comment from the spouse of an aphasic man:

> As a regular observer and frequent participant in his SLP sessions I felt the sessions were successful primarily in identifying what he could not do (Quann, 2002, p. 72).

---

[6]Avent and colleagues' questions could well be the comprehensive examination questions for graduate students working on a master's degree in communication disorders. And in fact, two of these researchers, Avent and Glista, ask their students to answer them—all of them—as an exercise (J. Avent & S. Glista, personal communication, 2006). I myself found that it is not an easy task.

The man, John Quann, was at a rehabilitation center after a stroke. His spouse, Eileen Quann, bright and curious and a true "John Quann expert," was knowledgeable about his former career at NASA before retirement. After observing a session in which he failed utterly at a sequencing task, she chose to recast it to reflect his interests, and the next day he successfully carried out the task with Eileen. Her sequencing task for John was far more demanding than the clinician's original one: She asked him to sequence the planets in order of their distance from the sun. (John also graciously pointed out that she had forgotten to include the now-demoted planet Pluto.) Family-as-expert cannot be discounted. We need to welcome their involvement. Communication counselors should ask families to partner in the specification and content of materials so that treatment tasks become personally relevant This inclusive approach will honor family members' expertise while simultaneously increasing their understanding of aphasia.

Consideration of some likely "counseling moments" is appropriate here. Some possibilities are included in Boxes 6.7 and 6.8. Box 6.7 focuses on concerns of persons who experience the disorders; Box 6.8, on concerns of families. Such "counseling moments," of course, can arise at any time, but most are particularly relevant for the rehabilitation center setting and for clinical intervention that may follow it.

## After the Rehabilitation Center

Box 6.9 completes Avent and colleagues' list of perceived needs relating to the end of time spent in the rehabilitation center, or perhaps when health insurance benefits tend to run out for communicatively impaired persons who required only outpatient services. Note that the tenor of the questions has changed. Now it focuses on getting on with life. An important source of useful answers to this list of questions and many additional ones is *The Aphasia Handbook*, a handbook developed at Connect, the pioneering British center for persons with chronic aphasia and their families. Its American version is available through the National Aphasia Association (Sarno & Peters, 2004). This is an important sourcebook, and communication counselors are urged to make it available to their clients and families.

## Box 6.7 "Counseling Moments" with Individual Clients Expected to Improve/Stabilize

The following comments from adult clients with communication disorders define clinical scenarios that result in specific "counseling moments." For each scenario, decide whether the "counseling moment," together with the requisite response, is something that is within your scope of practice. If you feel it is not, then answer from that perspective. If you decide it is within your scope of practice, answer from that perspective. (These example "moments" have some overlap with those for parents and children, as listed in Box 5.3. Some also are repeated in Box 6.8, for family/partner issues.)

"Funny thing . . . I got kinda lost in our own house yesterday."

"I know . . . what's wrong, but my kids—no way."

"I could live with this laryngectomy if I was sure I wouldn't get cancer again."

"No f-f-f-food. Why? Why?"

"My friends don't call me or come over any more."

"I know why . . . Speech . . . here (points around room) . . . good. You listen. Home, family, no! Family: 'Do your homework!' but just listen? Forget it!"

"But the bundles on the tarrapoi, say buddy . . . wagerstola."

"What's wrong with me? I know it—can't say it."

"It's all my fault. I messed up. Me! My fault!"

"I hate these hearing aids! Number one, I don't think I need them. If people spoke up, all would be fine. Number two, there is so much noise when I *do* wear them. Number three, they make me look old and unattractive!"

"Why does everyone act like there's something wrong with me? I know I have this trouble walking (points to left leg), but I don't even know why I come to see you! I'm just fine with my thinking."

**Box 6.8 "Counseling Moments" with Families and Partners of Persons Expected to Improve/Stabilize**

The following comments from partners and families define clinical scenarios that result in "counseling moments" specific for this counseling clientele. Perform the same exercises as outlined for Box 6.7.

"If I could just get my mother to come to spouse group, I think a lot of things would fall into place."

"I keep trying to tell my dad that he's got to stop working in the garden when it's so hot. I worry about him all the time."

"Jake got really angry at me last night. I just couldn't figure out what he wanted."

"I think I understand about aphasia, but this seems to be lost on our teenagers."

"Ever since the accident, I keep wondering when the bad dream will be over and Cassie will be her old self again."

"It's all my fault. Stuff like this happens all the time and messes up everything I do."

"I wish I could figure it out. Nothing like this ever happened to me before. I suppose it is just one isolated instance, and I shouldn't worry, right?"

"It makes me feel terrible that I have to lie to him so I can get him back to the nursing home without a scene and a tantrum. The only way I can get him into the car is to tell him we're going shopping or something, and by the time he gets back there, he forgets and it's okay. But I feel like a hypocrite."

"I have no time for me anymore."

The final counseling moment here is somewhat different. What do we do about family members who speak for their communicatively disordered member? Here is a scenario related to that problem:

Clinician (To Brian, the person with aphasia): "Well, Brian, did you have a busy weekend?"

Loretta (Brian's wife): "We sure did. All of the children and grandchildren cam over for a barbeque on Saturday, and Sunday we went to the movies after church."

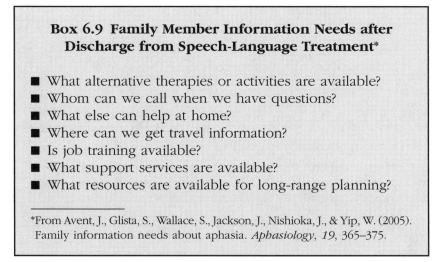

**Box 6.9 Family Member Information Needs after Discharge from Speech-Language Treatment\***

- What alternative therapies or activities are available?
- Whom can we call when we have questions?
- What else can help at home?
- Where can we get travel information?
- Is job training available?
- What support services are available?
- What resources are available for long-range planning?

\*From Avent, J., Glista, S., Wallace, S., Jackson, J., Nishioka, J., & Yip, W. (2005). Family information needs about aphasia. *Aphasiology*, *19*, 365–375.

Videotapes and DVDs also are beneficial. One such video, "Picturing Aphasia," was made by an artist interested in "exploring the limits of different forms of communication" (McWreath, 2006). The result is an illuminating documentary about aphasia and its effects on affected persons and families that can speak to them straightforwardly, through interviews and accurate, sensitive illustrations that augment and embellish them. Other relevant video tapes and websites are listed at the end of the chapter.

### *Living Well with Disability*

Without doubt, aphasic people can regain many communication skills after formal rehabilitation. But then the emphasis for communication counseling changes. The challenge for people with aphasia, or other disorders characterized by the likelihood of clinical improvement, is to begin the task of learning to live with disability. In her novel *Birds of a Feather* (2004), Jacqueline Winspear gets it just about right. Her heroine, Maisie Dobbs, is talking to Dr. Dene, an expert in rehabilitation of soldiers wounded in World War I:

> MAISIE: Tell me, Dr. Dene, if you were to name one thing that made the difference between those who get well and quickly and those who don't, what would it be?

> DR. DENE: Well, if I were to name one thing it would be acceptance.

MAISIE: Acceptance? But doesn't that stop the injured or wounded from trying to get better?

DR. DENE: In my opinion, acceptance has to come first. Some people don't accept what has happened They are stuck at the point of the event that caused the injury.

Maisie then asks Dr. Dene how people "get over" being stuck.

DR. DENE: I would say it is threefold. One is accepting what has happened. Three is having a picture, an idea of what they will do, when they are better, or improved. Then in the middle, is a path to follow. (p. 221)

From *Birds of a Feather* by Jacqueline Winspear. 2004. Penguin Press. Reprinted with permission.

Helping to set the "path to follow" is the initial counseling task after rehabilitation. As families and individuals begin to live into their futures, a distinctive counseling role is to help guide acceptance and acknowledgment in ways that permit and encourage living successfully and fully, despite communication problems. The goal is to fit the disability in, not get over it. The following poem addresses this goal well.

### The Cure

We think we get over things.

We don't get over things

Or say, we get over the measles but not a broken heart.

We need to make that distinction.

The things that become a part of our experience never become less a part of our experience.

How can I say it?

The way to "get over" a life is to die.

Short of that, you move with it.

Let the pain be pain, not in the hope that it will vanish

But in the faith that it will fit in.

Find its place in the shape of things

And be then not any less pain but true to form.

Because anything natural has an inherent shape

And it will flow towards it.

And a life is as natural as a leaf.

That's what we're looking for.

Not the end of a thing, but the shape of it.

Wisdom is seeing the shape of your life

Without obliterating (getting over) a single instant of it.

—Anonymous

Communication counselors also are urged to read Carole Pound's article "Dare to Be Different: The Person and the Practice" (2004). Pound writes from her dual perspectives as an SLP and as a person who has learned to live with chronic pain. Box 6.10 describes her particularly well-informed beliefs about appropriate clinician behavior.

---

### Box 6.10 How to Act as a Clinician Counselor*

- Act as a reference point.
- Act as a guide.
- Act as an advocate.
- Act as an interpreter.
- Help enable the aphasic client to feel like a person instead of a patient.
- Balance your professional expertise and confidence with listening and exploring "therapist naiveté" (issues of which you have little or no knowledge).
- Train other rehabilitation team members to be skilled conversation partners.

---

*Modified slightly from Pound, C. (2004). Dare to be different: The person and the practice. In J. F. Duchan & S. Byng (Eds.), *Challenging aphasia therapies*. New York: Psychology Press.

Although the course of change is toward improvement, it is both unpredictable and slow. Accordingly, both affected persons and their families should continue to engage in positive, disciplined behaviors designed to promote change and growth, for virtually the rest of their lives. For communicatively disordered persons, this can mean continuing to participate in therapy, or for many aphasic persons, helping others by participating in research projects designed to further current understanding of language disorders. Volunteering to be of service to others often is a meaningful activity as well. Commitment to full living may mean getting healthier, getting closer to one's children and grandchildren, taking more time to relax in a mindful way, learning things one never had time for before, and so forth. The following examples describe ways that two different aphasic persons chose to get on with life:

My friend Roger Ross,[7] who had very significant aphasia, demonstrated the benefit of positive disciplined behavior. Every morning of his life after his stroke, he read for an hour, moving from simple aphasia-friendly text early on to a point years down the road when he could once again manage his favorite fiction writers, as well as the political science works and current affairs books that had always been his love. Roger read much more slowly than before his stroke, a fact of his aphasia that he acknowledged and accepted. His efforts and illustrate growth and change in chronic communication problems. Such growth involves a willingness to work to change what makes personal sense to change and to be curious about how change occurs. It also involves willingness to make peace gracefully with what cannot be changed. Ross, for example, could have easily worked on his writing, as writing was his clear communicative strength. He chose not to do so, arguing that it took time away from what was more important to him: talking better and reading more efficiently.

---

[7]Roger Ross is his real name—he forbade the use of initials or pseudonyms, saying he was who he was and working to improve the lot of persons with aphasia. Roger Ross's inspirational video tape for aphasic persons is available through the University of Arizona Department of Speech, Language, and Hearing Sciences.

Another aphasic friend, LC, lived fully as well. But he did it differently—he just got back to his exuberant life as he had lived it before his stroke. LC also had very significant aphasia. When he realized that his golf game had barely been touched by his stroke, he returned to playing at least once a week. A particular joy for him was playing with strangers at a public course and managing not to reveal his language problem: "Those old guys . . . how about that? They didn't . . . Me? Not talkin' much." He also had at least one weekly lunch with friends. He went to plays and movies and took long trips in his car. He delivered Meals on Wheels, and he volunteered as a guide at a hospital. When I asked him how could provide directions around the hospital when his speech was so littered with paraphasias and difficult to understand, he smiled: "I don't talkin'. Nothing wrong in my wheat, seat, feet—I take 'em there."

Other aphasic people and their families have described this graceful making of peace in various ways:

It is a good retirement—just not quite the one we planned.

> Spouse of an aphasic woman, whose
> stroke occurred immediately following
> their very carefully planned retirement

I would say we are contented and lead a good life. But it is a different contentment and a different life.

> Spouse of an aphasic man

My own journey to "stroke-land" was different from any journey I'd taken before, but it was worth all the effort because I learned to laugh at myself and to trust myself. Before the stroke, I wouldn't have been able to see a brain attack as an opportunity for growth, but it gave me the chance to delve deep inside myself and find that I was tougher than I thought possible. (Perez, 2001)

Aphasia? I don't think about it anymore. (Ross, 2002)

> (This statement comes, paradoxically,
> from the video tape Ross made to
> inspire other persons with aphasia.)

Doing what needs to be done and what feels right for each individual—whether it is continuing to participate in aphasia groups, getting back to an exercise routine, taking a course in gardening or moving on, letting go—takes time. It cannot be rushed. Many people with aphasia report that it took longer than a year before things start seeming bright again. (See Holland, 2006, for more detailed discussion.)

A word of caution: Clinicians often have biases about what ought to happen or how it should happen. Biases are pernicious and often hard to recognize, but such "shoulds and oughts" are unacceptable in clinical contexts. A client with chronic aphasia who says "enough!" (or perhaps "more!") is to be respected and supported, even when we think we would make a different decision.

## Groups and Group Counseling

A major instrument in the clinician's counseling toolbox for chronic phases of disorders characterized by clinical improvement or stabilization is group intervention. Group treatment in general is the subject of very useful books by Elman (revised edition, 2007) and Pound, Parr, Lindsey, and Woolf (2000). Both sources provide many ideas about activities for groups, as well as how they should be organized and conducted. In the context of counseling, an important concept is that groups offer unique opportunities for individuals and their families to learn from each other and for people to come together in the powerful process of socializing once again.

The goals of groups are much more dependent on clinicians' counseling skills than on their more straightforward language intervention skills. Nevertheless, groups also serve as convenient practice sites for the activities that may be learned in individual sessions.

Groups are appropriate places for exploring and undertaking some of the exercises of positive psychology, in some cases slightly modified for use by persons with communication disabilities. Some such adaptations for use with groups (or with individual clients) are presented later in the chapter. Group work frequently is the catalyst for shaping the early steps in coming to grips with how life may be changed by the physical, behavioral and communicative consequences of the disorder. For families, the same goals of learning to be a part of society again also are foremost. The same counseling issues and approaches also are appropriate. Therefore, family groups pose similar challenges for communication counselors.

## Group Leadership Skills

Of the essential group leadership skills, one of the most important is the familiar "being a good listener." Listening involves leaving space for mulling over what has been said. It also means respecting the fact that in many instances, answers actually lie with the asker and not in the quick response of the answerer. A curious fact is that group silence, although relatively common during a session, may be construed as even more oppressive than one-on-one silence, so that the session leader may find it even harder than usual to count to 15 or 20 before responding. Leading an aphasia group in the process of developing coherence is particularly difficult. My own tendencies to respond quickly and with superficial consideration have been effectively reduced through my observation that if I hold my counsel long enough, someone else in a group situation (aphasia group or otherwise) usually will say what I am thinking. It helps to remember this while waiting out group silence, or while attempting to facilitate talk among group members.

Self-discipline is a related skill. Because clinicians are so-called normal speakers, they need to be wary of dominating the group interaction, or of attempting to direct it to ensure that all goes well. Self-control, sensitivity, and tact all are involved in making it possible for all group members to have floor time, and opportunities to participate to their own level of satisfaction. The central issue for counselors is being able to relinquish control comfortably. Although Roger Ross ran at least three highly successful groups entirely on his own, he refused to allow clinicians to help him with those groups or even to attend them. Clinicians tend to "take over" and "spoil it," he said (R. Ross, personal communication, discussed in Holland, 2007).

In facilitating aphasia groups, a special responsibility that relies on counseling skills is acting as a "communication broker." It is almost an art to interpret one aphasic group member's somewhat unintelligible communication to other group members who also have aphasia. Clinicians must be prepared to make mistakes while brokering and to learn to laugh at them, confident in the knowledge that laughter is an extremely important part of successful clinical intervention.[8]

As mentioned earlier in relation to rehabilitation centers, supported communication is another technical skill essential to successful communication counseling. Teaching its concepts to family members, however, is equally a clinical skill, a counseling issue, and an art. Box 6.11 contains some of the principles of supported communication, as outlined by Kagan (1998).

---

### Box 6.11 Principles of Supported Communication*

| To facilitate comprehension: | To facilitate speaking: |
| --- | --- |
| Supplement speech with pictures, objects, and written words or phrases | Encourage total communication; accept any modality used |
| Use natural gestures and drawings to augment speech | Provide relevant pictures, objects, and/or writing for client to use |
| Modify speech when appropriate, by slowing down, emphasizing key words, pausing at natural places | Allow extra time for speaking |
| Allow extra time for processing | Model use of total communication strategies |
| Signal speaker change with gaze or natural gesture | Facilitate sharing floor time |
| Signal topic change through use of total communication | Facilitate topic change when conversation lags |
| Confirm client's understanding | Resist "speaking for" another to the extent it is possible to do so. |

*Modified from Kagan, A., & Gailey, G. (1993). Functional is not enough. Training conversation partners for aphasic adults. In A. Holland & M. Forbes (Eds.), *Aphasia treatment: World perspectives* (pp. 199-225). San Diego, CA: Singular Publishing Group.

---

[8]For a thorough discussion of this and other useful notions, see Simmons-Mackie (2004).

Although it is clearly possible to train these skills one on one, teaching and practicing them in group settings are particularly effective. More examples can be shared, and for family members, learning these precepts also involves learning more about aphasia and its effects on others' lives. A useful supplement, not only for aphasic families but also for other health care professionals, is the set of guidelines provided by Holland and Halper (1996). Supported communication taught in partner group settings provides an excellent opportunity to facilitate peer role models and shared experiences as well. Although supported communication principles have been developed with aphasic persons in mind, they are applicable across the range of communication disorders associated with likelihood of improvement (with appropriate modification) as well.

An additional benefit of supported communication is that it can help adults with communication disorders to develop behaviors that help to put their non-impaired conversation partner at ease, thereby enhancing communication interaction. These skills are particularly useful for encounters with strangers or occasional interactants. Like supported communication itself, group therapy seems an ideal setting for learning them. Box 6.12 provides some suggestions for ways in which aphasic persons may help conversation partners, with the goal of improving interpersonal interaction.

## Individual Counseling

Communication counselors can have an equally viable role in one-on-one work with persons with communication disabilities. Each of the issues presented for group work can have a starring role in individual therapy as well, including the importance of sharing floor time, and attempting to achieve interactional parity.

One particularly pertinent issue, delicate and difficult to frame, stands out in individual work with adults. The concepts of shared expertise and aiding clients to develop resilience, identity, and self-efficacy seem at odds with traditional SLP-A concepts of feedback and external reinforcement. Arguably important in work with children, the use of the judgmental "Good" in its many instantiations, or the dismissive "Not quite—let's try again" in its various forms, can be toxic in work with adults. Judgmental comments about

---

**Box 6.12 For the Post-Stroke Client:
Helping Others to Help You**

1. Carry a card that explains your problem and what helps you to communicate better. For example:

   My name is Lester Breivold. I had a stroke, and can't talk very well. Please be patient with me. I do much better when the other person is patient. I have a pen and notepad, and I may ask you to write a few words to help me sometimes.

2. For clients who are able to learn such a message, it should be spoken as well. For example:

   I am Lester Breivold. I had a stroke. Speaking is difficult. Please be patient with me. I'll help you if I get stuck.

3. Learn what works to facilitate interactions. Ask for the help you need. For example:

   - Ask for repeats.
   - Ask partner to slow down.
   - Ask for the word to be written.
   - Ask interactant to look at you.

4. Put the interactant at ease with body language, smiles, and other indicators of good will.

---

adult clients' performance of clinical tasks probably undermine rapport and mutual respect.

Consider the effect (and the psychological cost) of telling Mr. E, a previously successful and articulate trial lawyer, that his attempt to say the word *cat* (or even *misdemeanor*) was "terrific." He knows it was not "terrific"—in fact, he is painfully aware that the word he produced was barely recognizable. For this client, pointing out what was *wrong* with his attempt may be less damaging because it is honest feedback concerning his everyday speech. Wording and content of feedback should be carefully considered for each situation. Box 6.13 presents some alternatives that reflect mutual expertise, are consistent with active positive responding, and do not damage identity.

---

### Box 6.13  Some Alternatives to "Good talking, Mr. Jones"

■ "I'm thinking that sounds a lot better—what do you think?
■ "Great, I think you got it. Did you, for real?
■ "If you're okay with that, so am I. Do you think the family will understand?"
■ "You know what? I don't think your kids will get that."
■ "Sometimes trying again helps—let's see if it helps you here!"
■ "Why don't you check to see if your message got through?"

---

## Some Positive Interventions for Counseling after Stroke

This section presents four activities from the positive psychology interventions described in Chapter 2 that have been adapted for use with stroke and spouse groups. Chapter 8 provides some coherent models for counseling workshops that are designed to build optimism and resilience in a systematic way, and exercises like these appear there, too.

### Identifying and Using Signature Strengths

Taking the VIA survey (described in Chapter 2 and available at www.authentichappiness.org) is beyond the skills of many persons who have language and communication problems after stroke. However, it is relatively easy to adapt the principles of the VIA for use as the basis for a group discussion, as follows:

> After the importance of using character strengths is intro-
> duced, each group participant is given a set of color-coded
> cards with one of the 24 character strengths written on each
> (e.g., strengths of wisdom and knowledge on green cards,
> strengths of transcendence on purple, and so on). All cards
> should be in the same order (*not* determined by color code)
> to facilitate use by readers and nonreaders both. The group
> leader reads each card aloud and asks the participants to

decide if the strength is "like me," "not like me," or "not sure," and then to place the cards on one of three stacks labeled YES, NO, and ??, respectively. When all 24 cards have been considered, participants go through their YES cards again, looking for the five that are most like them. These become the basis for exploring character strengths and virtues, what the color coding means, and so forth. Some possible illustrative questions follow:

- Are your five top cards all the same color? What does it mean?
- What does it mean if they are not?
- Was it easy to find cards that describe you? Did you have more than five?
- Which category makes the biggest of your stacks? (like me, not like me, not sure)
- From your "like me" stack, pick the one that describes you best. How did that strength help you most when you had a stroke?

This activity can be used with family groups as well, without the prompts by the group leader, and in an overall less tightly constrained form. For both groups, the relevant follow-up activity is to use one of the top five strengths during the next week, and making the experience the basis for the next week's discussion.

### A Good Thing Happened

"A Good Thing Happened" is an adaptation of the "Three Good Things" exercise (which can be used in its original form with partners and families). The concept embodied in this exercise is useful as a focus for group interaction or as an individual conversation topic. The clinician provides a personal example first and then asks each participant to tell of one good thing that happened during the week, using principles of supported communication to evoke the incidents, where necessary. All are written down for participants to study. Then the clinician uses his or her own example as the stimulus for the question "What did I do to bring it about?" Again, answers are supported and written. The only *wrong* answer is

"I didn't do anything—it just happened." That is the answer that everyone gets to challenge. For example:

> CLIENT:  Real good chocolate cone yesterday.
>
> CLINICIAN:  How did you bring that about?
>
> CLIENT:  Dunno . . . happened.
>
> CLINICIAN:  Not true! Did you decide when you saw the Häagen-Dazs store? Did you ask Mabel to get it? What?

The point of this exercise is to provide practice in taking responsibility not only for the bad things that happen in life but for the good ones as well. This is not always easy and in itself constitutes an excellent discussion topic.

### Positive Consequences of Stroke

The example provided in Box 6.3 was an unplanned moment of high positivity. It also is possible to engineer such moments. This exercise probably works best with people who have been living with their impairments for some time. It also may serve as a useful introduction for a new member of a group, particularly if the older members have practiced it before, and take the lead in sharing their answers with the new member. It is equally appropriate for stroke people or families. The stimulus topic can be presented as follows:

> "We spend a lot of time thinking about the problems that result from stroke. It's important to talk about them, but it is also a good idea to see if anything at all good came out of the stroke."

The clinician can provide examples such as the one from Box 6.3, but much simpler examples are acceptable as well.[9]

---

[9]One client said: "My daughter now calls us every weekend." My own favorite is from an inspirationally positive aphasic man: "I got a handicapped sticker for my car."

### *Gratitude Visit*

Families and affected persons are encouraged to work together on planning and carrying out a gratitude visit, as outlined in Chapter 2. In addition, however, an appropriate form of the post-stroke gratitude visit is to direct the visit to someone who has been particularly helpful in since the stroke—that is, someone who has made the adaptation process easier.

### *Stroke and Successful Living*

This is just a brief smattering of ideas, and more are presented in Chapter 8, along with exercises for increasing resilience and optimism. One underlying theme of such interventions is that attempting a working balance of a "pleasurable life," an "engaged life," and a "meaningful life" is a privilege to be enjoyed by everyone, including persons whose abilities have been compromised by an unexpected event. The exercises should serve as a reminder that the path to authentic happiness, even for the disabled, is really a two-way path. It is not just receiving gifts, cards, and letters from friends, but giving or sending them; not just getting one's communication supported by others, but helping others to be at ease in the presence of a communication disorder; not just learning to laugh again, but perhaps learning to make others laugh. Such considerations are part of the larger picture of successful living, with or without disability. My severely aphasic friend CR provides a final example: CR took a group of his good friends out to lunch each year on the anniversary of his stroke, to celebrate his continued survival in their company.

## Conclusions

This chapter has focused on stroke and its aftermath. Nonetheless, almost all of the concepts, principles, and exercises presented here can be applied in counseling and coaching for the other disorders with progression toward improvement/stabilization. Translation for application to those other disorders may involve careful consideration of other causes, specific facts of the disorders, and attributes of their treatment, but the principles and the issues remain largely the same: the concepts of building resilience and optimism, focusing on strength, telling stories, and sharing the expertise apply to the gamut from presbyacusis to TBI. It is part of the "whole catastrophe."

This chapter ends with a sensitive poetic description of aphasia and its effects on language

Aphasiaa

His signs flick off.

His names of birds

and beautiful words—

eleemosynary, fir, cinerarium, reckless—

scattering over linoleum.

His thinking won't

venture out of his mouth.

His grammar heads south.

Pathetic his subjunctives; just as pathetic

his mangling the emphatic enclitic

he once was the master of.

Still, all in all, he has

his inner weather of pure meaning,

though the wind is keening

through his Alps and his clouds hang low

and the forecast is "Rain mixed with snow,

heavy at times."

"Aphasia" Copyright 2004 by Vijay Seshadri. Reprinted from The Long Meadow with the permission of Greywolf Press, Saint Paul, MN

# References

Avent, J., Glista, S., Wallace, S., Jackson, J., Nishioka, J., & Yip, W. (2005). Family information needs about aphasia. *Aphasiology, 19*, 365-375.

Avent, J., Glista, S., Wallace, S., & Johnson, D. (2006). *What families want to know about aphasia: A survey study*. Manuscript submitted for publication.

Berger, P., & Mensch, S. (1999). *How to conquer the world with one hand and an attitude*. Merrifield, VA: Positive Power Publishing.

Douglas, K. (2003). *My stroke of luck*. New York: Macmillan.

Elman, R. (Ed.). (2007). *Group treatment of neurogenic communication disorders: The expert clinician's approach* (rev. ed.). San Diego, CA: Plural Publishing.

Helm-Estabrooks, N. (2002). Cognition in aphasia: A discussion and a study. *Journal of Communication Disorders, 35*, 171-186.

Hinckley, J. (2006). Finding messages in bottles: Living successfully with stroke and aphasia. *Topics in Stroke Rehabilitation, 13*, 25-35.

Holland, A. (2006). Living successfully with aphasia: *Three variations on a theme. Topics in Stroke Rehabilitation, 13*, 44-51.

Holland, A. (2007). The power of aphasia groups: Celebrating Roger Ross. In Elman, R. (Ed.). (2007). *Group treatment of neurogenic communication disorders: The expert clinician's approach* (rev. ed.). San Diego, CA: Plural Publishing.

Holland, A., & Beeson, P. (1993). Finding oneself following stroke. A reply to Brumfitt's "Losing one's sense of self following stroke." *Aphasiology, 7*, 581-583.

Holland, A., & Fridriksson, J. (2001). Management for aphasia in the acute phases post stroke. *American Journal of Speech-Language Pathology, 10*(1), 19-28.

Holland, A., & Halper, A. (1996). Communicating with individuals who are aphasic. *Topics in Aphasia Rehabilitation, 2*, 37-34.

Holland, A., & Ramage, A. (2004). Learning from Roger Ross: A clinical journey. In J. F. Duchan & S. Byng (Eds.), *Challenging aphasia therapies*. New York: Psychology Press.

Kagan, A. (1998). Supported conversation for adult with aphasia: Methods and resources for training conversational partners. *Aphasiology, 12*, 816-830.

Kagan, A., & Gailey, G. (1993). Functional is not enough. Training conversation partners for aphasic adults. In A. Holland & M. Forbes (Eds.), *Aphasia treatment: World perspectives* (pp. 199-225). San Diego, CA: Singular Publishing Group.

Mayer, T. (2000). *One handed in a two-handed world* (2nd ed.). Boston: Prince-Gallison Press.

McCrum, R. (1999). *My year off: Recovering life after a stroke*. New York: Broadway Books.

National Institute of Mental Health. (2006). *Depression and stroke fact sheet*. (Available at www.nimh.nih.gov.)

Peach, R. (2001). Further thoughts regarding management of acute aphasia following stroke. *American Journal of Speech Language Pathology, 10*, 29–36.

Perez, P. (2001). *Brain attack: Danger, chaos, opportunity, empowerment*. Johnson, VT: Cutting Edge Press.

Pound, C. (2004). Dare to be different: The person and the practice. In J. F. Duchan & S. Byng (Eds.), *Challenging aphasia therapies*. New York: Psychology Press.

Pound, C., Parr, S., Lindsay, J., & Woolf, C. (2000). *Beyond aphasia: Therapies for living with communication disability*. Bicester, UK: Winslow.

Quann, E. (2002). *By his side: Life and love after stroke*. Highland, MD: Fastrack.

Reivich, K., & Shatté, A. (2002). *The resilience factor: Seven essential skills for overcoming life's inevitable obstacles*. New York: Broadway Books.

Robey, R. (1998). A meta-analysis of clinical outcomes in the treatment of aphasia. *Journal of Speech Language and Hearing Research, 41*, 172–187.

Sarno, M. T., & Peters, J. (2004). *The aphasia handbook* (USA ed.). (Available through the National Aphasia Association, www.aphasia.org.)

Shadden, B. (2005). Aphasia as identity theft: Theory and practice. *Aphasiology, 19*, 211–224.

Seshadri, V. (2004). *Aphasia*. Saint Paul, MN: Graywolf Press.

Simmons-Mackie, N. (2004). Just kidding: Humor and therapy for aphasia. In J. F. Duchan & S. Byng (Eds.), *Challenging aphasia therapies*. New York: Psychology Press.

*Stroke Connection*. A publication of the American Stroke Association. (Available through www.strokeassociation.org; first year is free.)

*Stroke Smart*. A publication of the National Stroke Association. (Available at no cost through www.stroke.org.)

*Topics in Stroke Rehabilitation (2006). Consumer comments, control and communication, 13*, 1.

Wender, D. (1989). Aphasic victim as investigator. *Archives of Neurology, 46*, 91–92.

Winspear, J. (2004). *Birds of a feather*. New York: Penguin.

## Selected Websites and Videos on Stroke and Its Consequences

Adler Aphasia Center: www.Adleraphasiacenter.org

American Stroke Association, a division of the American Heart Association: www.strokeassociation.org

Aphasia Hope Foundation: www.aphasiahope.org

McWreath, J. M. (2006). Picturing aphasia. Video tape. (Available at www.aphasia.tv.)

National Aphasia Association: www.aphasia.org

National Stroke Association: www.stroke.org

Ross, R. (2002). Living successfully with aphasia. Videotape. (Available from the University of Arizona Department of Speech, Language, and Hearing Sciences. Tucson AZ, 85721)

## Chapter 7

# COMMUNICATION COUNSELING WITH ADULT CLIENTS AND THEIR FAMILIES FOR WHOM EXPECTED PROGRESSION IS TOWARD DETERIORATION

*M*ost communication counselors eventually encounter some clients with disorders that are not expected to change for the better and for which the best outcomes are maintenance of the current level of impairment and function for as long as possible. Such disorders are collectively referred to here as *disorders of downward progression* (in contrast to the disorders discussed in Chapter 6, which typically show improvement and upward progress). They include Parkinson's disease (PD), amyotrophic lateral sclerosis (ALS), Huntington's disease (HD), the variants of corticobasilar and cerebellar degeneration, supranuclear palsy, and, except for the few reversible ones, the entire range of dementias. These disorders worsen over time despite the best medical and behavioral therapies. They probably reflect a greater challenge to communication counselors than most of the other disorders discussed in this book; not only is dissolution of speech, language, swallowing, and, in some cases, cognition a concern, but also end-of-life issues appear.

As might be expected, depression is common among people who have these disorders as well as their families. A prevailing myth is that persons with dementia often are spared; the possibility of depression disappears, however, only after a dementing person has experienced major deterioration. For SLPs, the challenge of disorders of downward progression is somewhat mitigated by the fact that we are only infrequently the central counselors. Nevertheless, our counseling role is important and our responsibilities are unique. Box 7.1 presents some "counseling moments" for practice.

The disorders of downward progression also present challenges to the practice of positive psychology and to the development of hope and resilience. Nonetheless, what follows is not a rehearsal of despair, or even of merely coping; rather, numerous ways to make the most out of life, despite the conditions that signal its end, are suggested.

The chapter focuses on two quite distinct classes of disorders —one predominantly motor, the other cognitive. They are amyotrophic lateral sclerosis (ALS) and dementia, broadly defined to include a spectrum ranging from Alzheimer's disease (AD) (probably the most prevalent) to primary progressive aphasia (PPA) (possibly the most clearly relevant for communication counselors). Following the pattern of previous chapters, their salient counseling characteristics are discussed first.

## Amyotrophic Lateral Sclerosis

The motor neuron disease amyotrophic lateral sclerosis (ALS), or Lou Gehrig's disease, as it is popularly known, is progressive and invariably fatal. Both upper and lower motor neurons are ultimately involved, and patients lose the ability voluntarily to move their arms, legs, and the muscles involved in speaking and swallowing. Some recent work also suggests that persons with ALS may experience alterations in cognition as the disease progresses (Rippon et al.,

**Box 7.1 "Counseling Moments" with Families, Affected Persons, and Staff in Extended Care Facilities**

The following comments from families, affected persons, and staff define different clinical scenarios in extended care facilities. Decide whether the resulting "counseling moment," along with its response, is something that is within your scope of practice. If you feel it is not, then answer from that perspective. If you decide it is within your scope of practice, answer from that perspective.

**For families:**

"We live a life of isolation since the dementia started to get worse. We have no friends and no social life."

"I keep trying to tell my dad that he's got to stop working in the garden when it's so hot. After all, he has Mom to take care of, and he needs to be healthy. I worry about him all the time."

"It's really getting worse every day. I hardly sleep, I am losing weight, I have no energy or ambition, and I am wondering if its worth it to keep on trying . . . "

"I'm worried about the kids being around him. Is multiple sclerosis contagious?"

"I know I am a worrier, but I have a lot of trouble remembering names, and I get very distracted when there is too much noise. I keep thinking I'm getting Old Timer's Disease."

"I'm not getting any help from his children, and I simply can't manage him at home anymore."

"We've been worrying about Mom ever since Dad died a few years ago. It's only getting worse. She seems so fragile and failing. Her memory is going, and last week, her neighbors called to say she was wandering around, lost. The fact that we live over an hour away is really scary. What do you think we ought to do?"

**For persons with the disorders:**

"The doctor tells me I have Lou Gehrig's disease. But I really don't understand what that will mean for me. You have been very helpful with my swallowing. Now can you send me to a good website so I can get more information?"

"I feel like my mind is dissolving." [from a patient with PD]

"It's really getting worse every day. I hardly sleep, I am losing weight, I have no energy or ambition, and I am wondering if it's worth it to keep on trying . . . "

"I want to die."

"I know I should be practicing those exercises with you today. But I'm down. I have the feeling I brushed my own teeth for the last time this morning." [from a patient with non-bulbar ALS]

**For staff:**

"It sure would be nice if somebody had some ideas about making this place work better."

"I really go nuts when Mrs. Sertnus keeps saying, 'Help me!' She only wants attention, you know."

"If we can't figure out some way to get Mr. Finchley to eat, he's gonna end up with a plug, or dead!"

2006). Sensory abilities are not affected, and control of eye muscles appears to be intact in even well-advanced ALS. The preservation of eye movement makes it possible for many persons with ALS to use augmentative systems based on eye movement long after the disease has progressed significantly.[1] Ventilation sometimes is used to enhance breathing, but the usual cause of death in ALS is respiratory failure. Although the projected lifespan after its onset typically

---

[1]Insight into the world of such persons can be developed by reading Jean-Claude Beauby's book *The Diving Bell and the Butterfly* (1998), written only by use of eye movement and the help of his speech therapist. This disorder was locked-in syndrome resulting from stroke.

is 3 to 5 years, and ALS is most likely to occur in middle age, there are frequent exceptions. For example, the physicist Stephen Hawking, arguably the most famous ALS survivor alive today, was diagnosed in his early 20s and currently is in his sixth decade of life, communicating very effectively with a sophisticated augmentative device and living a full, if wheelchair-bound life.

The National Institute of Neurological Disorders and Stroke (NINDS) notes on the ALS page of the NINDS website that 90% to 95% of persons with ALS appear to have contracted the disease at random and have no clearly associated risk factors. The remaining 5% to 10% of persons with ALS appear to have inherited it, some from a specific genetic defect, which in the future may provide clues to the possible cause of ALS-associated neuronal degeneration and death. Although much current research is attempting to isolate the cause of ALS, to understand the mechanisms involved in its progression, and to provide effective treatment, no clear answers yet exist to help affected persons and their families to deal with these issues.

Furthermore, only one FDA-approved drug for the treatment of ALS—riluzole (Rilutek)—currently exists (see the NINDS ALS website). The drug does not cure ALS or reverse existing damage; however, it does appear to reduce (but not eliminate) some further neuron damage by decreasing the release of the neurotransmitter glutamate. Riluzole also appears to retard progression of dysphagia, and to extend the time before a patient requires ventilation. Because of its specific relationship to swallowing, riluzole is of particular significance to communication counselors involved with persons with ALS and their families.

Although ALS can have its earliest manifestations in any muscle group, a substantial number of affected persons have reported initial difficulty in speaking or swallowing or in problems such as choking or drooling. Even early on, persons with this form of ALS often have the telltale sign of tongue fasciculations. This presentation is known as bulbar ALS, and although dysarthria and dysphagia eventually develop in all persons with ALS, bulbar presentation provides early opportunities and challenges for beneficial and, to some degree, prophylactic intervention by SLPs in both direct treatment and counseling.

The opportunities reside in helping people with ALS and their families to develop proactive management strategies both for dysphagia, which will inevitably worsen, and for dysarthria, which will do the same. Clinicians provide this help by direct suggestions and techniques for "holding the line" as long as possible concerning management of glutition and nutrition, providing direct therapy for its distinctive mixed dysarthria, and helping the affected person and family to choose the most appropriate form of communication augmentation and then providing practice in its use.

The challenges for counseling come about in how we forecast the worsening. Helping the ALS person and his or her significant others to realize and deal with the fact that worsening will occur requires the clinician's counseling skills. Decisions concerning the use of ventilators and tracheotomies become central and therefore are major counseling concerns.

Nevertheless, persons whose ALS is initially bulbar can benefit from early speech-language pathology intervention, just as those with lower or upper extremity problems can benefit from early physical or occupational therapy. SLPs are most likely to encounter clients whose ALS had initial lower extremity expression only later in its course, but because SLPs still can make substantial contributions to managing problems of maintenance and change, the earlier their involvement, the more proactive help they can provide.

The central issues, then, for communication counseling concern the deterioration of function over time in swallowing and speaking, and maintaining quality of life despite it. Part of the problem is how to cope with the erosion of skills, but an equally salient concern is how to make the most of life under such circumstances. These issues are taken up later on.

## The Dementias

Management of the spectrum of dementias frequently requires different regimens of medical care, depending on the specific diagnosis. However, the generic label *dementia*, a "wastebasket" term for a number of conditions, is used here. This is primarily because, once the curable and treatable dementias have been eliminated, the basic issues for communication counselors (as opposed to medical personnel) do not appear to require the fine-tuning of more explicit labels. For example, for persons whose dementia is of indeterminate cause and for those who are presumed to have Alzheimer's disease (AD), there will be few differences in counseling needs.[2]

Most dementias are not in themselves life-threatening. Persons with dementia may live a decade or more after diagnosis and typically die from another condition that may be hastened by the aging process itself, rather than by the dementia. Dementia can be an indirect cause of death, however, as a result of changes in cognitive status that result, for example, in increased poor judgment or in indifference to safety or nutrition.

A plethora of websites address Alzheimer's disease, the most common form of dementia. A few examples, with extensive links to others, are listed at the end of the chapter. These sites describe extensive ongoing scientific research devoted to this problem. Investigators currently are learning much more about the changing neurology and progression of AD. For the rare familial form of early-onset AD, the inheritance pattern has been found to be autosomal dominant, with gene mutations on chromosomes 1, 14, and 21. Additional evidence indicates that persons who inherit one or two copies of the APOE e4allele, as opposed to copies of e2 or e3, on chromosome 19 appear to be at increased risk for AD. Beyond this, however, no clear-cut genetic linkages to AD are known. Other, possibly more environmentally mediated causes of AD also remain unclear, and pharmaceutical agents such as tacrine (Cognex), donepezil (Aricept), and rivastigmine (Excelon) have only limited effectiveness in slowing progression in a small number of people. Even the sources of neuritic plaques and neurofibrillary tangles that are AD's signature pathology remain elusive.

Few other dementias are as well explained as AD. Although progress is constantly being made in understanding, for persons who become demented and for their families, much about the dementias remains as baffling and perplexing as it was nearly two decades ago. SLP-As who work with dementing persons are urged to study the comprehensive text by Bayles and Tomoeda (2007).

---

[2]Primary progressive aphasia (PPA) may be an exception, and some of that disorder's unique issues are discussed separately later, when pertinent. Another exception may be multi-infarct dementia. Many of these patients know their families, their own histories, and identity until nearly the end, and this makes a great difference to caregivers.

Such matters are at the heart of dementia's counseling issues. Few pharmaceutical or direct behavioral interventions are effective; tremendous family burden often persists for long periods of time; and heart-wrenching decisions must be made concerning placement and management. Fortunately, the counseling responsibilities for the dementias typically are spread out over a number of helping professions. But because deteriorating communication is an ever-present signal of cognitive decline, the role we play is substantial.

Similar to traumatic brain injury (TBI) in this regard, language problems in dementia seldom exist as the central concern. Difficulties with memory, executive functioning, or more general cognitive functioning occupy that role. Rather, language is the medium through which persons with dementia express their other cognitive problems and make them manifest to their significant others. Also as with TBI, for clinicians the result is a subtle shift away from interventions directed at improvement of speech, hearing, and language. Instead, intervention often focuses on environmental manipulations that support and bolster language and memory. It also includes helping to reduce the effects of these bewildering problems on others in the dementing person's environment. A major difference from TBI is the downward progression of dementia. Once again, maintaining function for as long as possible and slowing the rate of decline are goals with persons who have dementia, rather than working to effect lasting improvement, as is the case with TBI.

The issues of ventilators and tracheotomies for persons with advanced motor speech disorders have been mentioned previously. But it seems clear that the counseling issues in dementia are in synchrony with those that arise with use of feeding tubes and other technologies that can possibly extend life. We should be ready to discuss the pros and cons of such interventions with families of dementing persons as well. Again, listening to families, helping them to clarify the issues, and providing valid information to aid in their decision-making all require counseling skill.

## The Concept of Ambiguous Loss

People and families facing disorders of downward progression share what family therapist Pauline Boss calls "ambiguous loss" (1999). Boss defines *ambiguous loss* as loss that remains unclear, indeterminate, and unresolved for some period of time, with a lingering lack of closure and clarity. Ambiguous losses get frozen in time, making it difficult, if not impossible, for grieving and other methods for handling outright loss to be fully exploited. Communication disorders such as those discussed here are not alone as examples of ambiguous loss. Many other medically determined illnesses, such as slow-growing malignant tumors, also can be cited as examples of ambiguous loss.

One of Boss's two major types of ambiguous loss has particular resonance for the disorders of downward progression. Boss characterizes this type of ambiguous loss as that involving "goodbye without leaving" (1999, p. 45).[3] Because of the centrality of disturbed communication and cognitive processes in disorders of downward progression, *goodbye without leaving* is an apt metaphor for people who still are alive but who cannot communicate in their usual style or who have changed in some fundamental ways. Boss's concern is primarily for families in these circumstances, but it seems obvious that people who suffer from ALS or any of the dementias in early stages also feel their own ambiguity in loss of self. They doubtless experience pain when they confront the fact that they are indeed leaving without goodbye. Here, Boss's metaphor, along with her suggestions for handling ambiguous loss, is explored as a counseling focus.

"Goodbye without leaving," in Boss's view, is a most painful form of loss. For persons with disorders such as ALS, the loss becomes more apparent to others as communication progressively fails. The source of the loss in ALS is largely physical. One of the counseling responsibilities with such patients and their families is to provide and then to encourage the use of strategies and devices to augment dwindling skills or to serve as alternative forms of communication—that is, to prevent "goodbye without leaving" for as long as possible. Counselors can help families in strategy development, as in the following example:

> Gideon, a retired man with progressive dementia, has for some time consistently begun his day with a walk to his favorite

---

[3]Boss terms the other type of ambiguous loss "leaving without goodbye." Such losses occur with the disappearance of persons with whom it was not possible to share farewells, such as birth mothers of adopted persons or soldiers who are missing in action.

neighborhood café. He is well known there by both other neighborhood denizens and the café staff, and he always orders the same thing. As his dementia develops, Phoebe, his wife, has become increasingly nervous about this routine and seeks to curtail it. Phoebe is concerned primarily with Gideon's safety, but also about embarrassment for both of them.

A short-term solution involves creative problem-solving. For example, perhaps a visit to the café staff, for Phoebe to explain Gideon's new problems and provide guidelines concerning how to handle them, may be of benefit. When Gideon leaves the house, it may be worthwhile to follow him a couple of times to assure Phoebe that he is capable of making the trip alone. Concerning his time at the café, a helpful intervention may be to explain his condition to a few of his café buddies and give them a few suggestions for including him in their conversations.

This approach also is appropriate for persons with PPA, for whom a similar implementation has been well described and documented (Rogers, King, & Alarcon, 2000).

## As Loss Grows More Apparent

Once motor or cognitive difficulties substantially worsen, clinicians face a counseling dilemma related to shared expertise. Is it our responsibility to encourage communication once it becomes exceedingly laborious or, in the case of dementia, when communication becomes manifestly uninteresting to the communicator? Our profession recognizes implicitly that communication, maintained as long as possible, postpones "leaving" in the sense described by Boss. But for some people who live with the disorders of downward progression, communicating simply becomes too difficult, or consumes too much energy, or the person reaches a tipping point at which communicative attempts come to represent a loss of dignity and choice. When this occurs, then the matter is truly out of the clinician's hands. Strand (2003) describes this as an issue that places our beneficence—doing good for the patient—in conflict with his or her autonomy. The gifted clinician must seek a balance here, by asking and clarifying, and then backing off from encounters when the affected person chooses not to communicate.

As noted earlier, Boss's major concern is for families who witness and endure their loved ones who say goodbye without leaving. She provides many helpful suggestions for families with the uncertainties inherent in dealing with psychological absence in the face of physical presence. Following is a list of suggestions, adapted from her work, for communication counselors working with disorders of downward progression:

- Recognize no "right" way to cope with uncertainty.
- Reinforce behaviors that encourage physical activity and interaction with others.
- Encourage respite as necessary for tolerating ambiguous loss.
- Use humor as a coping mechanism.
- Guide families to harmonize with nature instead of attempting to master it. (Boss, 1999, pp. 114–116)

The following account of the course of ALS as experienced by a client of mine serves to provide affirmation that despite the disease, life can be lived to the end with purpose and dignity:

Mr. Luther had bulbar ALS. Soon after he was diagnosed, his wife of 50 years died suddenly of heart disease. The Luthers were childless, so Mr. Luther found himself almost alone in the world except for a sister who visited monthly and a small circle of friends. Mr. Luther, the president of a small technology company and an engineer by training, took his adversities in stride. He was a resilient person, with a passion for problem solving. Concerning his dysarthria, for example, he worked hard on developing marble-sized one-way valves to insert into his nasal passages, in hopes of reducing his increasing nasality. He could not use a standard palatal lift, so he invented one of his own, shaped like McDonald's "Golden Arches" and held in place by string and a button that stuck out of the corner of his mouth. Neither device worked, but he took great pleasure in creating them. (He also carried a plastic spray bottle, filled with his favorite wine, which he used liberally as his "best relief" both for moistening his dry mouth and for decreasing saliva.)

Frugal to a fault, as Mr. Luther's ALS worsened, he chose Magic Slates over other, more sophisticated communication device, cutting the slates in quarters not only so they would fit comfortably in his shirt pocket but because it saved money. He took great pains to have his affairs and his advance directives in place, making it clear to his neurologist that when he could no longer swallow, he wanted only palliative care. He also made it clear that he wanted only his sister to be with him at the end. That wish was respected.

Mr. Luther kept his autonomy until the end and accepted his impending death with grace and temperance. He said goodbye, and then made sure to leave soon thereafter.

## Positive Psychology and Disorders of Downward Progression

Does positive psychology have anything to offer? The answer is an unequivocal yes. The diagnosis of an inevitably fatal disease should not be translated immediately into "Abandon hope, all ye who enter here." Rather, it makes sense to help people with incurable diseases and their families to consider ways to live their remaining lives as fully as possible, and to help them and their families to proceed along the road of their ambiguous losses with grace and equanimity.

Joanne Koenig Coste has written a remarkably rich sourcebook for families and individuals involved in dealing with Alzheimer's disease. Her book *Learning to Speak Alzheimer's* (2003) has many implications not only for the other dementias but for most of the ambiguous losses discussed thus far. Koenig Coste names five basic tenets of habilitation, optimally applied all together in specific situations, summarized as follows:

- *Make the physical environment work.* Alter the environment in ways that help make the person feel safe, successful, comfortable, and free of distress.
- *Know that communication remains possible.* The emotions are more important than the word, and it is the emotions that need to be validated. When it's no longer possible to listen to the mouth, "listen" to the eyes.
- *Focus only on remaining skills.* Value the abilities that remain. Help the affected person to compensate without calling attention to it.

- *Live in the person's world.* Join the person in his or her current "place" or time, no matter when or where that may be, and find joy with the person there.
- *Enrich the person's life.* Create moments for success, eliminate potential moments of failure, praise frequently and with sincerity. Attempt to find joy wherever possible.[4] (Condensed and adapted from Koenig Coste, 2003, Chapters 6 to 10)

Koenig Coste, like Cynthia Kidder in Chapter 4, never uses the words "positive psychology" or "authentic happiness" in her book. Yet she has written an affirming and fulfilling book, jammed with good ideas and suggestions for living positively with Alzheimer's disease. Most expand on the tenets listed here. Also, like Kidder's, they have come from her own experience in living with the disorder. Communication counselors should encourage families and individuals with dementia to read such works, preferably as early as possible in the course of the disease, so that they can apply the ideas effectively. Most of the ideas, however, have significant implications for living in institutionalized settings as well.[5]

I know of Mark Reiman and his contribution to the ALS literature only because I encountered his ideas on the ALS Association website (www.alsa.org). An interview he participated in 8 years after his ALS diagnosis, and 4 years before his death, is a treasured resource. Very little additional information about him is available, but his words indicate that he was a caring, measured, and brave person. Following is a list of his principles, in greatly condensed form. In essence, they constitute the framework of the counseling approach presented in this chapter.

- Seek support.
- Hold fast to hope.
- Be active in your own health.
- Realize that your life may have changed but that it's far from over. (Adapted from Interview with Mark Reiman, 1999)

---

[4]Dementia, particularly as it worsens, is likely to shrink the "pleasurable life" to the present, with perhaps only snatches of early past remaining and the future no longer contemplated. Thus, the affected person should be helped to make the most of it—to live his or her remaining life "in the moment."

[5]The transcript of a very informative interview of Koenig Coste by the *New York Times* in 2004 is available via googling "A Conversation with Joanne Koenig Coste.

# Listening to Mark Reiman: A Positive Communication Counseling Perspective

Reiman's (Interview, 1999) principles seem comprehensive enough to serve as the springboard for elaborating on some issues in counseling persons and families experiencing disorders of downward progression. In this section, each of his points is expanded upon from the perspective of communication counseling.

## Seek Support

At least early in the course of the disease, persons with disorders of downward progression can benefit from participation in groups in much the same way as for persons with post-stroke aphasia. The approach to group counseling outlined in Chapter 6 is readily applicable here.

Particularly for persons with dementia, however, group leaders will find that increased structure usually is necessary. In fact, for both group and one-on-one encounters, persons with dementia benefit from structure, constraint, and repetition, in contrast to aphasic persons, who appear to flourish with freedom from them. The primary goal for such groups should be psychosocially oriented, with provision of opportunities to engage as fully in life as possible under changing circumstances. To capitalize on strengths, an important consideration is that early memories probably are more intact than recent ones, and that lifelong patterns remain familiar as well, not only motor behaviors such as walking, or using the sounds of one's native language, but the lifelong habits of doing daily chores, of going to work, and of being responsible.

These realities can be the basis for highly rewarding group activities. In her important resource book *Care That Works* (1999), Zgola describes the Tea Group, a program for "difficult" [sic] residents of a long-term care (LTC) center in Ottawa, Canada, that has been in operation, despite different facilitators and members, for many years. Perhaps the goal of preparing and drinking tea is more appropriate to a committed tea-drinking country such as Canada; some adaptation may be in order for residents of the United States, where Starbucks rules. In any case, the Tea Group provides a constrained common ground, rich in habits and rituals of a lifetime, and conducted in a safe, supportive, respectful environment that exemplifies an effective model for groups whose members have dementia.

By contrast, groups for persons with ALS or other progressive motor disorders can further the agendas of keeping as healthy as possible and preparing for change, as well as providing psychosocial support and the sharing of strengths. Most of the positive psychology interventions from Chapters 1 and 8 are appropriate. Particularly for such groups, it is important to remember that for many participants, offering as well as receiving help is a benefit.

At least as important are partner, spouse, and family groups. The tremendous burden faced by significant others in living with and managing their partners' disorders of downward progression can be substantially influenced and lessened though group interactions. The "36-hour day" described by caregivers (Mace & Rabins, 2001) feels all too real. Caregivers need help to solve some of the problems they encounter in those long hours, as well as camaraderie and assurance that they do not bear their burdens alone.

Families of persons who have incurred strokes have similar problems, and approaches to their group counseling are similar. Using the questions in Boxes 6.4, 6.6, and 6.9, substitute the term *dementia* or *ALS* (or any of the progressive disorders), to appreciate their goodness of fit across the spectrum of these disorders.

It often is awkward and indeed disheartening for spouses of persons with PPA or the other disorders discussed here to attend groups with those whose partners have had strokes, because the courses of the disorders are fundamentally different. This is in marked contrast with the parent support groups discussed earlier, in which parents often can profit from contact with parents of children whose problems differ from those of their own children. From this perspective, it makes sense to include PPA families in dementia groups, rather than in stroke groups.

It's also possible for persons to seek and receive support without joining a formal group. The Internet once again can be useful, and social institutions such as churches can be particularly helpful. Communication counselors need to familiarize themselves with programs available in their communities. For example, in Tucson, where I live, several churches provide support and respite for families with dementia, and my neighborhood has a model program for assisting elderly and infirm persons to remain in their own homes for as long as possible.

## Hold Fast to Hope

Reiman's statement of hope (1999) is well nuanced and balanced by the acknowledgment implicit in his other principles. This is not the "cockeyed optimism" that was cautioned against earlier. Rather, holding fast to hope is simply recognizing the importance of maintaining a positive attitude, even in the face of great odds. It fits well with two of Boss's tenets for managing ambiguous loss, particularly her comment that there is no right way to cope with uncertainty, and with her goal of guiding families to harmonize with nature (and its course), rather than trying to master it (Boss, 1999). Counselors who work with disorders of downward progression must be particularly careful not to dash the hope and optimism of clients, who may need to see things differently from their clinicians. We not only have no answers to give to them but in fact do not know how we ourselves may react in similar situations.

## Be Proactive in Health Care

Reiman reminds us that wellness is not only for the well, it can also be an attitude and a stance for the chronically, even desperately, ill.[6] This is not a contradiction but an affirmation about living a "pleasant life," an "engaged life," and a "meaningful life" for as long as possible. Holman and Lorig (2004) and Lorig and colleagues (Lorig & Holman, 2003; Lorig, Hurwicz, Sobel, Hobbs, & Rittler, 2003 have spearheaded a self-management approach to chronic diseases such as arthritis and diabetes that has permitted affected persons to be proactive and committed to seeking wellness in the midst of their disabling conditions. John Argue, an expert in movement and voice who has Parkinson's disease, has created a comprehensive positive exercise plan for other affected persons (2000). The spirit of the Lee Silver-

---

[6]As a breast cancer survivor, I can attest to this. During my extended period of radiation therapy, I never skipped a day of playing racquetball with Jane, my usual partner. In fact, during that time I played so well that both of us considered my radiation might be supplemented with doses of Kryptonite or some such mythical source of power. When the radiotherapy stopped, however, I returned to my previous mediocre form, and Jane and I realized that she had been unconsciously going easy on me during those weeks. Nonetheless, being able to play at all, particularly with a caring partner, truly buoyed my spirits and my sense of engagement in life.

man Voice Therapy (LSVT) regimen lies in its allegiance to energizing and wellness (Fox, Morrison, Ramig, & Sapir, 2002). The National Center on Physical Activity and Disability (NCPAD) is committed to appropriate exercise programs for persons with deteriorating as well as stable disabling conditions and features on its website well-designed and tested programs for ALS and other degenerative motor disorders (www.ncpad.org). NCPAD also supports Arkin's ElderRehab program (Arkin, 1999). This program uses volunteers as aides in an effective physical exercise-language enrichment program for persons with dementia. The specifics of this program are available in a detailed resource manual (Arkin2005). Communication counselors need to be aware of such programs and encourage their use.

Throughout this chapter, it has been difficult to avoid use of the term "patient" to refer to these irreversibly impaired ill clients. To support a philosophy of wellness, this term is also best avoided in clinical practice. It is important for communication counselors to embrace the notion of wellness for their clients despite disability, and to encourage wellness not only for disabled adults but for affected children and their families as well.

## Life May Be Changed, but It Is Not Over

The concept of living each day to its fullest has been emphasized throughout this book, and now it takes us back to the philosophy of Zorba the Greek, described in Chapter 1. "Full catastrophe living" most likely eludes people who are well into middle or late stage of their disorder, but it should not elude their partners and families. In this culture at least, wives are not expected to emulate their spouses' deterioration. Suttee, the practice of widows throwing themselves on their husbands' funeral pyres, is banned in India, where it once was common. It certainly should not be practiced even metaphorically in the presence of chronic illness. A particularly important point in this context is that respite from responsibility and maintaining humor are strong antidotes to the burdens of giving care. Not only do caregivers benefit; so do the persons for whom they are caring.

When finally convinced by her clinician and her children to take a weekend trip to San Francisco with a friend, and to leave the caregiving for Mr. Y, who had moderate dementia, in the hands of her very capable daughter, Mrs. Y went reluctantly. She returned 3 days later, refreshed from three nights with 8 hours of uninterrupted sleep, renewed by finally seeing the renovated Ferry Building about which she had heard so much, and by the gourmet meals she ate as she revisited her favorite restaurants. But there were other benefits as well. Mrs. Y learned that her daughter was a fine surrogate caregiver for short trips, that traveling with a friend produced worthy companionship and certainly more enjoyable shopping than she had ever experienced with Mr. Y, and finally, that he barely noticed her absence, and thrived on his daughter's doting. Mrs. Y is making plans for another trip 3 months hence.

This story was told in an AD partner group. The group had heard Mrs. Y's previous agonizing about every aspect of this trip and in fact had played a role in convincing her to go. The group members magnanimously refrained from a chorus of "We told you so," possibly because she was testing the waters for most of them as well. They could now begin the process of making plans of their own, perhaps. This is the power of support groups, which are particularly helpful in promoting the concepts of living each day as fully as possible, rather than concentrating on dying.

## "Practice Your Greatest Freedom"

This section begins with Mark Reiman's (Interview, 1999) exhortation to "practice your greatest freedom." He went on to offer the following advice:

Choose to make this defining moment an opportunity for your greatest love, your greatest vision, courage, determination, and compassion. Surround yourself with positive people. (Interview with Mark Reiman, 1999, para. 4, #5)

There is perhaps no stronger, more positive message for persons with disorders of downward progression and their families.

In Chapter 3, Victor Frankl noted that "choosing one's way" is the greatest freedom afforded to human beings (Frankl, 1989). Reiman explicitly acknowledges its importance in relationship to his own life-threatening illness. How can communication counselors help their clients to hear such a message, to understand it, and to apply it to their lives?

This message is not for sissies. Nor is it a message that can be promoted as a viable possibility to persons who don't understand it, or who don't think they can adopt it. Nonetheless, it can be shared and discussed, preferably in groups, where opinions may differ and alternatives may be explored. As an exercise, re-read Reiman's or Frankl's statements; then check on who in the group believes this message, why it makes a difference to them, and what beliefs it is in conflict with (such as feeling victimized by one's disorder, or helpless in its presence). This message is one of life's most affirming ones, and even though not everyone can embrace it, everyone deserves a chance to consider it. Communication counselors can help to make that happen.

## Counseling in Long-Term Care Settings (LTCs)

Thus far in this chapter, the settings for intervention for the disorders of downward progression mostly have been home-based. That is, most of the clients and families who have the disorders have been presumed to be living at home. This is not the case for many such persons, particularly those with relatively slowly deteriorating disorders exemplified by significant dementia. SLPs are increasingly visible in LTC settings,[7] and audiologists are beginning, finally, to be seen there as well, where they have an important part to play in enhancing the quality of life for elders who can profit from amplification. As has been true of all of the settings discussed in this book, LTC settings also offer unique opportunities and challenges.

---

[7]LTC settings also may include group homes, assisted living centers, nursing homes, and special care units set up in nursing homes or in assisted living centers primarily for persons experiencing worsening dementia.

One major counseling issue of relevance here may be keeping these families to reach their personally most comfortable decisions concerning placement in an LTC setting. Clearly, communication counselors seldom are the sole sources for dealing with issues such as this, but they often have an important role to play, particularly if they have been involved with management of the dementing person when he or she was still at home. The counseling skills do not change, but the focus is on helping the family and, whenever possible, the person with the disorder, to make a decision that is right for them. Joanne Koenig Coste makes a critical comment: " . . . all families will do far better when the considerations of lifespan care are dealt with on the basis of realistic assessments, rather than on guilt" (Koenig Coste, 2003, p. 192). Finally, three principles, already referred to in this book, should remain foremost in counseling regarding long-term placement:

- The counselor's job is to provide options and encourage exploration of them.
- There are neither right nor wrong decisions. There are only decisions one can live with.
- Decisions should reflect the values of the affected person(s), not the counselor's.

As in rehabilitation centers, LTC facilities are becoming increasingly more likely to encourage staff to work as members of interdisciplinary teams, rather than to remain isolated in the traditional fiefdoms of nursing, occupational and physical therapy, social work, and speech-language pathology and audiology. As a result, SLP-As' counseling functions are likely to be modified as well. One important new role may be as a consultant to other staff members concerning disturbed communication and nutrition and what can be done about them. Typical in-service training sessions probably should center less on language in dementia and more on how to improve communication on site, through techniques that are taught to the staff in general, both for their own interactions with residents and to help reduce communication frustration for visitors, and on ways to promote nutrition. Some examples of LTC-centered activities developed by SLPs or occupational therapists (OTs) that address each of those issues are presented next. Many more are available; all involve counseling skills to promote the most effective implementation in often fairly inflexible settings.

## Improving Staff Communication with Residents

The important role of self-cueing and the use of cue cards in improving communication in LTC settings have been well documented (Bourgeois, Dijkstra, Burio, & Allen-Burge, 2007; Bourgeois & Hickey, 2007). Essentially, the process involves teaching staff to develop appropriate, situation-specific index cards that residents can be taught to read aloud and use to cue their behaviors. For example, a Certified Nursing Assistant (CNA) may be taught to help Mrs. T modify her repetitive questioning through the use of handwritten index cards:

### Pre-Teaching Scenario:

MRS. T:  Where are my dentures?

CNA:  I just told you 5 minutes ago that they are being fixed and will be back next Tuesday. [*This interaction may occur countless times daily.*]

### Post-Teaching Scenario:

MRS. T:  Where are my dentures?

CNA: The answer is on your card, Mrs. T. Read your card aloud.

MRS. T:  [*Reads*] "My dentures are being fixed. Back on Tuesday."

CNA: Great, Mrs. T. Your dentures will be good as new next Tuesday. Next time you need to know, look at your cards. [*This interaction may occur three or four times, but practice ultimately lessens the repetitive questioning.*]

The use of cue cards is a straightforward technique, simple to teach to staff. So where is the counseling involved? Communicating the method's value to the staff and demonstrating its effectiveness both require counseling skills. One facet is explicitly acknowledging the CNA's expertise. He or she probably has more knowledge of most of the residents than that possessed by the clinician-counselor. A recommended approach is to consult the CNA often, seeking partnership and demonstrating, rather than announcing, the counselor's own skills. In addition, it is wise to point out to CNAs how they may benefit from learning the approach, because it can make their jobs easier and more pleasant. Many more examples are provided in the work of Bourgeois and colleagues (2001, 2007), Koenig Coste (2003), and Zgola (1999) mentioned earlier, as well as by other writers of sourcebooks for working with dementia, such as Nissenboim and Vroman (2003). Although this book is not about management of dementia, it should be recognized that in LTC settings, the counseling roles of SLP-As often extend beyond family to other staff and support personnel.

## Improving Visitor Interactions with Residents

A comprehensive and readable booklet (Brush, 2002) is available to guide visitors in ways to improve their interactions with residents of LTCs. It is a good example of the extensive training materials available to improve daily life in LTCs. The material in this particular booklet does not need to be presented one on one; it easily stands alone. Counseling skills are involved in convincing senior staff of the value of such materials for families and indeed for anyone who interacts with residents. It offers a way to improve resident visits, by providing a common language and a consistent opportunity for enriching contacts for everyone. Making this happen is more likely if the SLP-A practices good counseling skills.

Finally, just as supported communication principles make sense for use with aphasia, they also are applicable with dementia. There is some overlap, to be sure, but some divergences as well. Small and colleagues' work in this area (Small, Gutman, Makela, & Hillhouse, 2003; Small & Perry, 2005) is especially instructive and applicable to both families and caregivers.

## Environmental Manipulations That Positively Affect Nutrition

A staff attuned to interdisciplinary collaborations can implement literally hundreds of environmental manipulations. The instigator may well be a communications expert, of course. Only one example is featured here, partly because it emphasizes the role of SLPs in managing nutritional issues and partly because, once again, counseling skills are not always directed at issues with residents or care providers. Here, they are employed in influencing administrative decisions. "Counseling" is not what the communication counselor does with administrators. Nevertheless, approaching such issues with counseling skills is highly recommended if changes are to be implemented.

Brush, Meehan, and Calkins (2002) described an approach to management of insufficient nutrition for residents of an LTC facility. These investigators chose a few residents who were not getting adequate nourishment, and who were candidates for mechanical feeding support (e.g., placement of feeding tubes). Before the experiment began, they measured participants' weight and their caloric intake, and observed their eating habits and behaviors. Two environmental manipulations followed. The first was to increase the color contrast between the table setting and the plate (both were neutral, perhaps making it difficult for residents to discern their plates and their food). The second was to increase the illumination available in the dining room setting, to increase visibility overall. During the intervention, Brush and colleagues measured caloric intake, and at the end, they weighed the participants again. Once the intervention was in place, food intake was increased; as a result, participants gained weight

Where were counseling skills involved? First, to obtain permission to conduct the experimental intervention, Brush and her colleagues (2002) needed to convince the administration of its value. Then it was necessary to ensure that the changes were implemented. Thus, the outcome measure was increased intake, and by freeing CNAs of their responsibilities for urging the residents to eat, these projects led to better use of personnel time. These types of messages resonate with staff and administration alike.

## The Problem of Dysphagia

Dysphagia may occur with many of the disorders covered previously (e.g., stroke). For many persons with swallowing disorders, substantial psychosocial issues, such fear of choking, embarrassment over difficulty in eating unusually textured foods, and prolonged length of time required for eating, are increasingly recognized. Such issues may predispose dysphagic persons perhaps to eat alone, rather than engaging in the social interactions that accompany mealtimes. (For a cogent overview, see Martino, 2005.) These problems pull dysphagia into mainstream communications counseling and do not necessarily require specialized counseling expertise. Nevertheless, such concerns truly demand our attention.

When dysphagia is life-threatening to a person whose disorder is inevitably getting worse, as in ALS, or when the affected person may not understand all the issues, as in dementia, the placement of feeding tubes becomes both a compelling issue for families and a great challenge for communication counselors.

Irwin (2006) noted that SLPs often play an important role not only in counseling but also in advising others who may be providing counseling about the placement of feeding tubes. Irwin was specifically discussing persons whose condition had deteriorated to dependence on feeding tubes for maintenance of life, but many of his points are relevant to persons with advanced ALS as well. In light of limited data on effectiveness of feeding tubes for preventing aspiration (Chouinard, Levigne, & Villeneuve, 1998; Dharmarajan & Unnekreshnan, 2004; Finucane, Christmas & Travis, 1999) SLPs face dilemmas about how to advise family members, even when advance directives are already in place. (Irwin notes a startling finding by Shega and colleagues (2003) indicating that 36% of physicians would place a feeding tube at a family's request, despite advance directives to the contrary.) Other studies indicate that both SLPs and physicians often have incomplete information about the limited effectiveness of feeding tubes (Carey, 2005; Conti, 2003).

Listening to families and helping them to clarify such issues, providing them with significant and valid information to aid them in making decisions regarding feeding tubes, and the like are counseling functions. As Irwin (2006) suggests, however, appropriate counseling requires professionals who have a predominantly rehabilitative outlook to shift their outlook to a palliative one. This means essentially shifting attention toward an attitude of "active total care of patients whose condition is not responsive to curative treatment," as defined in 1990 by the World Health Organization (WHO) (WHO definition of palliative care, 2001). Box 7.2 provides the WHO's complete definition of palliative care.

---

**Box 7.2 Dimensions of Palliative Care***

- Affirms life and regards dying as a normal process
- Neither hastens nor postpones death
- Provides relief from pain and other distressing symptoms
- Offers a support system to help patients live as actively as possible until death
- Offers a support system to help the family cope during the patient's illness and in their own bereavement

---

*From World Health Organization definition of palliative care. (2001). In C. F. von Gunten, F. D. Ferris, R. K. Portenoy, & M. Glajchen (Eds.), *CAPC manual*. (Online publication.) New York: Center to Advance Palliative Care. Retrieved April 2, 2006, from http://64.85.16.230/educate/content/palliative caredefinitions/WHO

---

## Are All LTC Facilities Created Equal?

Both good LTC facilities and barely passable ones are certified, despite their differences in philosophy, quality and range of services, and outlook. Communication counselors may well find themselves in the role of providing information to families about the quality of the institutions they are considering, listening to their concerns, and guiding them in their choices. Koenig Coste provides sensible guideline for families to follow. The list of guidelines gets longer as the need for services increases from assisted living to special dementia units. Koenig Coste stresses that few LTC facilities, even at the assisted living level, will meet all expectations, but it is nonetheless worthwhile to consider these guidelines from a personal standpoint, looking for the facility that comes closest to the family's ideal. Her basic guidelines for assisted living appear in condensed form in Box 7.3.

An excellent approach to LTC has been developed by The Eden Alternative, a community-based model that focuses on maximizing quality of life for both residents and workers in LTC facilities.

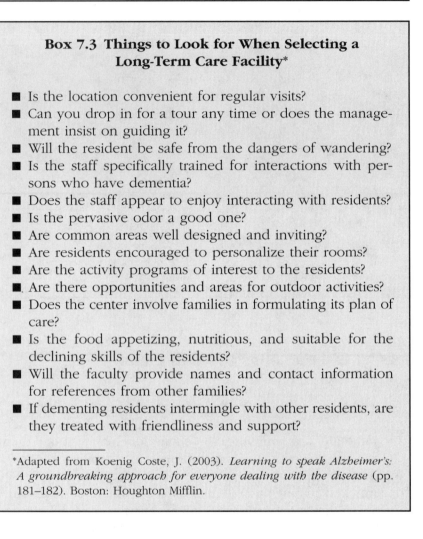

**Box 7.3 Things to Look for When Selecting a Long-Term Care Facility***

- Is the location convenient for regular visits?
- Can you drop in for a tour any time or does the management insist on guiding it?
- Will the resident be safe from the dangers of wandering?
- Is the staff specifically trained for interactions with persons who have dementia?
- Does the staff appear to enjoy interacting with residents?
- Is the pervasive odor a good one?
- Are common areas well designed and inviting?
- Are residents encouraged to personalize their rooms?
- Are the activity programs of interest to the residents?
- Are there opportunities and areas for outdoor activities?
- Does the center involve families in formulating its plan of care?
- Is the food appetizing, nutritious, and suitable for the declining skills of the residents?
- Will the faculty provide names and contact information for references from other families?
- If dementing residents intermingle with other residents, are they treated with friendliness and support?

*Adapted from Koenig Coste, J. (2003). *Learning to speak Alzheimer's: A groundbreaking approach for everyone dealing with the disease* (pp. 181–182). Boston: Houghton Mifflin.

According to The Eden Alternative website, this model is dedicated to creating "coalitions of people and organizations that are committed to creating better social and physical environments for people." From the perspective of positive psychology, it is difficult to imagine a more appropriate LTC facility than one grounded and trained in Eden Alternative principles, presented in Box 7.4. Such LTC facilities are flourishing across the United States. SLP-As who are considering working in extended care settings may find these principles useful as a gauge against which to judge an environment in which they wish to work.

## Box 7.4 Eden Alternative Principles*

1. The three plagues of loneliness, helplessness, and boredom account for the bulk of suffering among our Elders.

2. An Elder-centered community commits to creating a Human Habitat where life revolves around close and continuing contact with plants, animals and children. It is these relationships that provide the young and old alike with a pathway to a life worth living.

3. Loving companionship is the antidote to loneliness. Elders deserve easy access to human and animal companionship.

4. An Elder-centered community creates opportunity to give as well as receive care. This is the antidote to helplessness.

5. An Elder-centered community imbues daily life with variety and spontaneity by creating an environment in which unexpected and unpredictable interactions and happenings can take place. This is the antidote to boredom.

6. Meaningless activity corrodes the human spirit. The opportunity to do things that we find meaningful is essential to human health.

7. Medical treatment should be the servant of genuine human caring, never its master.

8. An Elder-centered community honors its Elders by de-emphasizing top-down bureaucratic authority, seeking instead to place the maximum possible decision-making authority into the hands of the Elders or into the hands of those closest to them.

9. Creating an Elder-centered community is a never-ending process. Human growth must never be separated from human life.

10. Wise leadership is the lifeblood of any struggle against the three plagues. For it, there can be no substitute.

---

*From The Eden Alternative. (2002). *Our 10 principles*. (Available at www.edenalt.com. Reprinted with permission.

## Conclusions

As supported by the content of this chapter, counseling and coaching are at least as much an attitude and a state of mind as they are a set of skills brought to bear on a problem of interest. A major concept presented in Chapter 3 is the importance of identifying detrimental personal attitudes and maintaining respect for those whom we counsel. Attitude seems pervasive in relation to the disorders focused on here. Perhaps this is because our roles with these disorders are less clear and, particularly with dementia, have only recently been recognized as important.

Irwin (2006) was astute in describing our optimal role with dysphagia in late-stage dementia, or with ventilator placement in late-stage ALS, as palliative, rather than rehabilitative. His observation should be extended, however, to include *all* disorders of downward progression: Palliation is the indicated approach in each of these disorders. Accordingly, communication counseling will be central to all of our interactions and engagements with affected persons, their families, and staff members of the facilities where they may ultimately reside.

Joanne Koenig Coste has had infinitely more direct experience with disorders of downward progression, or at least in dementia, than most people. Her earliest encounter with Alzheimer's disease occurred well over 30 years ago when her husband (somewhat older than she) was first suspected of having it, while she was pregnant with their fourth child. From her story, it appears that she embraced the disorder, accepting its challenges and its inevitable changes, and, on the death of her husband, moved toward it. Instead of closing the door on that chapter of her life, she found her life's work in learning more about Alzheimer's disease, as well as in sharing her personal experiences with others who find themselves in her same boat. Even today, her attitudes and her creativity remain intact, and she has not suffered the burnout reported by many people who work with these disorders. Whatever Koenig Coste's particular character strengths may be, certainly bravery and vitality must be high on the list.

Koenig Coste may well be the Johnny Appleseed of Alzheimer's disease, sharing her compassion, her ideas, and her knowledge with those who need it most, and carrying forward the wisdom she also has gained from others. It seems appropriate to end this chapter with her observations on how persons with dementia can best be supported to live well:

- Reminding and scolding me does not make me better, only sadder. When someone asks me questions about where I've been and who I've seen and what I did, and I can't retrieve that information, I feel stupid and unworthy.
- Trying to fill my brain with new ideas and new equipment and new data will not work. My brain is full. Not one speck of space is left for new information to find a seat. If the information can't go in, it can never come out again.
- Don't wish me out of reverie or worry about my silent times. I still have imaginative explorations to make, and dreams to dream. I have kisses to relive. I have a garden of memories before me , and everything is blooming simultaneously. Don't assume I am sad when I sit alone; most of the time it is the sadness on your face that brings sorrow to my heart.
- You can make me a part of this world only if you actively involve me, if your connection with me remains until the end. You must constantly reach out and touch me—physically, spiritually, emotionally.
- You are the conduit to my failing world, a world that has so many possibilities to be filled with laughter, a few shared tears, and memories (pp. 198–199).

> From *Learning to speak Alzheimer's: A ground-breaking approach for everyone dealing with the disease*, by Joanne Koenig Coste. 2003 Houghton Mifflin. Reprinted with permission.

These words apply to persons with all varieties of dementias and, perhaps with the exception of the second point, to all of the others whose disorders involve saying goodbye without leaving, as well.

# References

Argue, J. (2000). *Parkinson's disease and the art of moving*. Oakland, CA: New Harbinger.

Arkin, S. (1999). ElderRehab: A student-supervised exercise program for Alzheimer's patients. *The Gerontologist, 39,* 729–735.

Arkin, S. (2005). *Language enriched exercise for clients with Alzheimer's disease*. Tucson AZ: Desert Fitness.

Bayles, K & Tomoeda, C. (2007). Cognitive-communication disorders of dementia: Definition, diagnosis, & treatment. San Diego, CA: Plural Publishing.

Beauby, J.-C. (1998). *The diving bell and the butterfly*. New York: Vintage.

Boss, P. (1999). *Ambiguous loss: Learning to live with unresolved grief*. Cambridge, MA: Harvard University Press.

Bourgeois, M., Dijkstra, K., Burgio, L., & Allen-Burge, R. (2001). Memory aids as an AAC strategy for nursing home residents with dementia. *Augmentative and Alternative Communication, 17*, 196–210.

Bourgeois, M., & Hickey, E. (2007). Dementia. In D. Beukelman, K. Garrett, & K. Yorkston (Eds.), *Communication strategies for adults with acute or chronic medical conditions*. Baltimore: Paul H. Brookes Publishing.

Brush, J. (Ed.). (2002). *Ideas for a better visit*. Kirtland, OH: Ideas Institute.

Brush, J. A., Meehan, R. A., & Calkins, M. P. (2002). Using the environment to improve intake in people with dementia. *Alzheimer's Care Quarterly, 3*(4), 330–338.

Carey, T. S. (2005). Use of feeding tubes in the care of long-term residents. *North Carolina Medical Journal, 66*, 313–315.

Chouinard, J., Lavigne, E., & Villeneuve, C. (1998). Weight loss, dysphagia, and outcome in advanced dementia. *Dysphagia, 13*, 151–155.

Conti, G. (2003). Speech-language pathologists' role and knowledge levels related to non-oral feeding. *Journal of Medical Speech-Language Pathology, 11*, 15–31.

Dharmarajan, T., & Unnikrishnan, D. (2004). Tube feeding in the elderly; The technique, complications and outcome. *Postgraduate Medicine, 115*, 51–54, 58–61.

Finucane, T., Christmas, C., & Travis, K. (1999). Tube feeding in patients with advanced dementia: A review of the evidence. *Journal of the American Medical Association, 282*, 1365–1370.

Fox, C., Morrison, C., Ramig, L., & Sapir, S. (2002). Current perspectives on the Lee Silverman Voice Treatment (LSVT®). *American Journal of Speech Language Pathology, 11*, 111–123.

Frankl, V. (1989). *Man's search for meaning*. New York: Washington Square Press.

Irwin, W. (2006). Feeding patients with advanced dementia: The role of the speech-language pathologist in making end-of-life decisions. *Journal of Medical Speech-Language Pathology, 14*, xi–xiii.

Holman, A., & Lorig, K. (2004). Patient self-management: A key to effectiveness and efficiency in care of chronic disease. *Public Health Reports, 119*, 239–243.

Interview with Mark Reiman. (1999). (Available at www.als.com.)

Koenig Coste, J. (2003). *Learning to speak Alzheimer's: A groundbreaking approach for everyone dealing with the disease*. Boston: Houghton Mifflin.

Lorig, K., & Holman, H. (2003). Self-management education: History, definition outcomes and mechanisms. *Annals of Behavioral Medicine, 26*, 1–7.

Lorig, K., Hurwicz, M., Sobel, D., Hobbs, M., & Rittler, P. (2003). A national dissemination of an evidence based self-management program: A process evaluation study. *Patient Education and Counseling, 1*, 69–79.

Mace, N. L., & Rabens, P. V. (2001). *The 36-hour day: A family guide to caring for persons with Alzheimer disease, related dementing illnesses, and memory loss in later life*. Baltimore: Johns Hopkins University Press.

Martino, R. (2005.) Food for thought: Does what the patient thinks really matter? *Perspectives on Swallowing and Swallowing Disorders (Dysphagia), Division 13 Newsletter of the American Speech-Language-Hearing Association, 14*(4), 24–26.

Nissenboim, S. & Vroman, C. (2003). *The positive interactions program of activities for people with Alzheimer's disease*. Baltimore: Health Professions Press.

Rippon, G. A., Scarmeas, N., Gordon, P. H., Murphy, P. L., Albert, S. M., Mitsumoto, H., et al. (2006). An observational study of cognitive impairment in amyotrophic lateral sclerosis. *Archives of Neurology, 63*, 345–352.

Rogers, M. A., King, J., & Alarcon, N. B. (2000). Proactive management of primary progressive aphasia. In D. R. Beukelman, K. Yorkston, & J. Reichle (Eds.), *Augmentative communication for adults with neurogenic and neuromuscular disabilities* (pp. 305–337). Baltimore: Paul H. Brookes Publishing.

Shega, J, Hougham, Stocking, C., Cox-Hayley, D. & Sachs, G. (2003). Barriers to limiting the practice of feeding tube placement in advanced dementia. *Journal of Palliative Medicine, 6*, 885–893.

Small, J., Gutman, G., Makela, S., & Hillhouse, B. (2003). Effectiveness of communication strategies used by caregivers of persons with Alzheimer's disease during activities of daily living. *Journal of Speech, Language and Hearing Research, 46*, 353–367.

Small, J., & Perry, J. (2005). Do you remember? How caregivers question their spouses who have Alzheimer's disease and the impact on communication. *Journal of Speech, Language, and Hearing Research, 48*, 125–136.

Strand, E. (2003). Clinical and professional ethics in the management of motor speech disorders. *Seminars in Speech and Language, 24*, 301–311.

World Health Organization definition of palliative care. (2001). In C. F. von Gunten, F. D. Ferris, R. K. Portenoy, & M. Glajchen (Eds.), *CAPC manual*. (Online publication.) New York: Center to Advance Palliative Care. Retrieved April 2, 2006, from http://64.85.16.230/educate/content/palliativecaredefinitions/WHO.

Zgola, J. (1999). *Care that works*. Baltimore: Johns Hopkins Press.

## Websites

National Institute of Neurological Disorders and Stroke ALS webpage: www.ninds.nih.gov; follow links to "Disorders" and then "Amyotrophic Lateral Sclerosis"

ALS Association: www.alsa.org

Alzheimer's Association: www.alz.org

Alzheimer's Foundation of America: www.Alzfdn.org

National Center on Physical Activity and Disability: www.ncpad.org

National Institutes of Health SeniorHealth Health Information for Older Adults: www.nihseniorhealth.gov

# Chapter 8

# TEACHING RESILIENCE AND OPTIMISM TO FAMILIES AND CLIENTS WITH COMMUNICATION DISORDERS: SOME WORKSHOP FORMATS

Scattered throughout this book are suggestions for counseling moments and exercises that foster adaptation, growth, and the development of positive attitudes concerning communication impairments and their consequences. To this point, it has been assumed that they would be applied within the traditional formats for individual and group treatments in speech-language pathology and audiology. This penultimate chapter describes an additional model—short-term workshops specifically targeting the importance of resilience, optimism, and positive attitudes for persons who have communication disorders and their families, partners, and parents, as applicable. Some activities for these proposed workshops have been discussed in earlier chapters; they are revisited briefly in this new format. Others are presented here for the first time. Just as many of the previously described activities can fit into a short-term workshop model, the new ones can be used in more standard individual and group treatment sessions.

## Format and Background for the Workshops

The short-term workshops described here each consist of four sessions, one and one-half to two hours in length, spread over four consecutive weeks. In my experience, this time frame works well for the busy schedules of many clients and professionals, although other formats can be used. The activities can very easily be spread over more sessions (say, six) or over longer periods (say, meetings every two weeks), or perhaps concentrated into an all-day workshop. This last format precludes the advantage that spacing provides—namely, that participants have an opportunity to try out the material, report back, and make it possible for the facilitator to debrief or help to correct, if necessary. The workshops can also be considerably expanded. The suggested activities are not cast in concrete either. They are merely suggestions, chosen from a much wider array of potential activities, either because some have data to support their effectiveness or because in my own clinical practice they have been especially useful with persons who have communication disorders.

The workshops are designed for any number of participants. Although the frameworks for, say, 10 attendees would be more personalized than they would be for larger groups, the principles do not vary. For example, if the workshop is small, then during the first session everyone probably will be able to share experiences; this will certainly not be possible with 30 or more participants.

As mentioned in Chapter 4 in relation to group activities, workshops for parents of at-risk children probably can be broad, and families can learn from others with different problems quite successfully. But there is no inherent problem in directing a workshop toward a specific disability, such as autism or Down syndrome. The suggested reading lists and websites may vary with the focus topic, but little else. Workshops for older children and adolescents who stutter or who have incurred traumatic brain injury (TBI) probably should be disorder-specific, particularly if bonding and reaching out are to be emphasized. Severity of the disorder should provide guidelines as well.

Positively oriented workshops for adults and their families are different. There, my preference is for workshops to be disorder-focused. The rationale for this preference has been presented earlier in this book. Although the workshop principles do not differ, and in many cases, the activities also are similar, mutual support and bonding are less likely to be effective if persons with aphasia and right hemisphere brain damage (RHD) or TBI, or their families, participate in the same sessions, or when persons with dementia and those with disorders such as amyotrophic lateral sclerosis (ALS) are grouped. This is largely because the challenges of these disorders differ markedly.

This chapter provides communication counselors with an alternative framework for helping their clients begin to discern the benefits to be gained by practicing some of the principles espoused in this book. It is not a blueprint for conducting such workshops; it is merely a set of workable ideas. Neither are four sessions like these likely to change the course of anyone's life.[1] Nevertheless, such workshops may constitute the first step along a path. They can provide common ground for future counseling; they also can serve as the necessary stimulus for participants to follow through with self-directed activities such as reading and applying relevant, lay-oriented materials such as in Reivich and Shatté's book (2002), or involving themselves through the Authentic Happiness website (www.authentichappiness.com) or lay readings described earlier, or in taking the online courses based on the work of Reivich and Shatté. Again, the online courses can be accessed through www.reflectivelearning.com.

This chapter contains workshop outlines for parents of children with disabilities, and for families of adults who have incurred communication disorders. For the parent workshops, no particular disorder has been specified, in line with my belief that getting together parents of children who have different disabilities can be a plus.

For the family workshop, activities are focused on families (spouses, partners, children) of disabled adults, occasionally using

---

[1]In fact, it is not even particularly likely that at the end of the workshops, direct or potentially long-lasting effects will be found. In a workshop based on this model that I conducted with persons with acquired immunodeficiency syndrome (AIDS), supportive bonds were formed that have continued. But the real value is reflected in a comment made a year later by a member of the group, who told me that the workshop had been the impetus for a year of personal exploration and change (including breaking his previously unbreakable addiction to cigarettes) that was still ongoing.

some specific disorder as illustrative. Some topics and exercises for parents and family differ only in their details (where the devil has been said to reside), but some are unique to each target group. Nevertheless, the basic information can be generalized to other family or disorder groups, such as Parkinson's disease or Alzheimer's disease (AD), as well as to parent groups aimed at specific disorders such as autism or Down syndrome.

A review of communication counselors' preparation for conducting these workshops follows. Then the parent and family workshops are presented in detail. Finally, ideas concerning how they may be modified for use with adolescent stutterers and with persons with aphasia are explored. These latter workshop variations are described only briefly, owing to the overlap with the family and parent approaches.

## Workshop Preparation for Communication Counselors

If you are still reading this book, then it is obvious that it is a recommended text. Nonetheless, other very useful readings can help you prepare for conducting workshops of this nature. Many references from other chapters constitute excellent background material, particularly Seligman's *Authentic Happiness* (2002), Peterson's *A Primer in Positive Psychology* (2006), and Reivich and Shatté's *The Resilience Factor: Seven Essential Skills for Overcoming Life's Inevitable Obstacles* (2002).

Performance of at least one "dress rehearsal" of this workshop is recommended before implementation with the relevant group. A simple way to practice is with colleagues, or students, or even a group of persons with communication disorders or their families with whom you have had extensive and positive contact, and who can be counted on to provide constructive feedback. (Many of these willing "guinea pigs" will find the workshops interesting and useful in their own lives.)

The cardinal difference between workshops and more traditional group sessions is that workshops frequently attempt to teach new skills or to reach new understandings based on new learning. Accordingly, they typically incorporate information-giving, in the form of informal lecturing, as well as through interaction among the group's participants. These workshops are no exceptions. Nonetheless, even though new information is emphasized, the basic commitment to shared expertise should be respected. This means that group leaders must recognize the importance of their listening role as well as their talking one. Group leaders facilitate learning along with the experience of putting the concepts and the exercises into practice. The experiences and the group's discussion of them are central. It often is worth skimping on the informal lecturing for the sake of just jumping into it.

In many cases, the exercises for the parent and family versions will overlap. When they do not, both a parent and a family variant are provided. Of note, all of these exercises and homework instructions are presented as simply springboards for counselors' own creative adaptations. Incidentally, the terms *counselor*, *facilitator*, *leader*, and *communication counselor* are used interchangeably in this chapter.

# Week 1

As with classroom teaching, one of the leader's first responsibilities is to let the participants know what they can expect to learn and experience, and what is expected of them. The purpose of this initial session is to start that process, and to get participants acquainted with one another as they begin to share solutions and strengths and to provide support for one another.

## The First Activity: A Positive Start

An effective way to initiate these workshops is the "You at Your Best" example presented in Chapter 2. Box 8.1 contains a modification that has been used successfully for this purpose. It serves both as an experiential introduction to positive psychology and as an excellent first step in building new relationships. During the exercise, a lot of noise and laughter can be expected. It's important to point this out when it happens, and to expand on it in the general discussion, as described later on.

Following the sharing of stories, the group leader then asks a participant whose partner told a very good story to share it with

---

**Box 8.1 Week 1: You at Your Best—Workshop Format**

**Instructions:** Think of a time in your life when you were at your very best. Then write a brief description of the event and what you did that showed you at your best. It doesn't have to be a long description, perhaps just some notes on it. Limit yourself to 10 minutes for the entire exercise.

Now find someone you don't know in this room; go sit with that person, and tell each other your stories. This should take about 10 minutes.

---

the group. Depending on the time, the leader may ask two or three people to tell their partner's stories. Some good questions for initiating the general discussion include the following: "What strengths were you using?" "How else do you use that strength?" The facilitator may wish to mention that the group will explore the subject of such strengths more deeply later on.

Focusing this first discussion on the point that there is joy and laughter, however brief for most people, despite life's burdens, brings a lighter, generally positive note to the workshop experience. By contrast, imagine beginning a workshop for parents or families by asking people to share one significant problem faced by them or their child or aphasic family member—the tone would be quite different, with a much more solemn outcome. Seligman (2004) noted that our bad experiences are like Velcro in that they seem to stick to us; our positive ones slip away as if they were coated in Teflon. Putting one's best foot forward often is awkward for people because of the "Velcro effect," and is a good discussion point as well. Other discussion points may include the importance of sharing stories with others and how such sharing furnishes an interesting counterweight to the common tendency to focus on problems, rather than on successes.

### The Second Activity: Participant Introductions

The second activity of this session is to make sure that participants begin the process of learning to know each other. Participants are each asked to say why they are here, to introduce themselves briefly, and also briefly to describe their child or the family member. Depending on group size, such disclosure can be more or less detailed. The leader's initial job is to model the introduction in his or her own identifying comments and then monitor the time, provide organizing remarks, and finally summarize shared and unique experiences, common themes, and the like.

## Introducing Positive Psychology

The introduction to positive psychology should be as brief and as informal as possible. Chapter 2 provides a good starting place. It is useful to cast the information into a form that considers the questions "Why do some parents or families or individuals with aphasia seem to cope better than others?" and "What does it take to be resilient?" Then the facilitator can discuss the idea that the science of positive psychology examines questions like these and is beginning to provide some tentative answers. For example, the following abilities describe families or parents who do well:

- Understand the three paths to authentic happiness
- Know their strengths
- See alternatives
- Have an optimistic attitude, tempered by realism
- Know how to use, or to counteract, their explanatory styles
- Have "bounce back" and "muddle through" skills
- Know when and where to seek help

The goal is not to explain positive psychology in any depth but simply to let parents or families know that they will be learning some skills and techniques during the course of the workshop that will be useful in launching them in an affirming direction.

## The Third Activity:  Character Strengths/Virtues

The final activity of the first session is to participate in the card shuffle version of the character strengths and virtues activity described in Chapter 6. The version presented there was for use with aphasic adults, but it is easily adaptable here for parents or families as well. Some suggestions for group discussion after completion of this activity are given in Box 8.2.

---

**Box 8.2  Week 1:  Signature Strengths Card Shuffle—
Sample Discussion Questions**

- Are your five top cards all the same color? What does that mean?
- What does it mean if they are not?
- Was it easy to find cards that describe you? Did you have more than five?
- Which is the biggest of your stacks? ("Like me," "Not like me"?)
- From your "Like me" stack, which one describes you best?

**For parents:**

Did that strength help you since your child was born? How? Is it helping you now?

**For family members:**

Did that strength help you since your spouse's (or partner's or parent's) illness? How? Is it helping you now?

---

## Homework

Homework is an integral part of this workshop model. Homework helps to ensure that the ideas discussed during each session go beyond the session's confines to practical application at home. Reivich points out that homework provides an opportunity to take the ideas presented in a workshop for a "test drive" so that in subsequent sessions, it is possible to focus on what was successful and what was not (K. Reivich, personal communication, 2006).

It is a good idea to provide small spiral notebooks to participants so that they can record their experiences in doing the assignments. An alternative is to provide formatted assignment sheets that summarize the exercises and provide space for writing a summary of the experience. Box 8.3 describes the first homework task, a set of extensions of the "You at Your Best" activity. Workshop participants are asked to try to do at least one of these assignments, or perhaps more.

### Box 8.3  Week 1: Homework—Everybody at His/Her Best in the Everyday World

**Parent Version**

- Think of a time when you were at your very best with your handicapped child. Then write a brief description of the event and what you did that showed you at your best.
- Think of a time when your partner was at his or her very best with your handicapped child. Then write a brief description of the event and what he or she did.
- Think of a time when one of your other children was at his or her very best with your handicapped child. Then write a brief description of the event and what he or she did.
- Think of a time when your handicapped child was at his or her very best. Then write a brief description of the event, and what your child did.

Clearly, nobody will do all of these within a week. But they are important to think about. Try to write at least a few words for yourself (possibly to share with the group) about the first and last. Revisit the exercise as often as possible, if only in your thoughts.

**Family Version**

- Think of a time when you were at your very best with your disabled family member. Then write a brief description of the event and what you did that showed you at your best.
- Think of a time when your family member, since the disabling event, was at his or her very best with you. Then write a brief description of the event and what he or she did. Does it compare in any way with the person at his or her very best *before* the disabling event?
- Think of a time when another family member was at his or her very best with the disabled family member. Then write a brief description of the event and what he or she did.

> Clearly, nobody will do all of these within a week. But they are important to think about. Try to write at least a few words for yourself (possibly to share with the group) about the first two. Revisit the exercise whenever you need to.

(Different versions for parents and families are presented.) Even when they have not completed them, most participants report that they have at least thought about the assignments. (This also can be a subsequent discussion focus—that is, what makes the exercises hard for some people to do?)

The second homework assignment is to reconsider a strength that each participant has identified through the card shuffle exercise, and to use that strength in a new way during the week before the next workshop session.[2] This exercise, described in Chapter 2 in relationship to the formal VIA questionnaire, is easily adaptable here.

## Week 2

As will be the pattern for the rest of the workshop sessions, the second session starts by sharing the lessons learned and some of the experiences that occurred in carrying out the assignments. It is unreasonable to expect that all workshop participants complete all assignments, but some will. They will have stories to tell that are informative not only to other participants who did the assignments but to those who did not. Here is a good place to find out what may make exercises hard for some participants. It also is a good place to ask the "non-doers" (gently) if the experiences that any of the doers reported were useful to them. This is a time for story sharing, and as in the session that preceded it, the leader's role is to monitor time, to point out themes and so forth, and to summarize what the group members have discovered about themselves or others.

---

[2]As noted earlier, Peterson (2006, pp. 159-162) presents a long list of ideas concerning how to do this.

## Defining and Discussing Resilience

The second session then explores what resilience is, and why it is important to learn and practice resilience skills. This is a crucial point for parents who are raising challenging children, or for families who are living with a disabled adult. A handout for this session could be the list of characteristics of Vietnam prisoners of war who did *not* develop post-traumatic stress disorder as presented in Box 2.2. It is important to point out that becoming more resilient is possible; one's ability to bounce back, or to steer through, or simply to take life in stride is not immutable. Change and growth are possible.

There are a lot of resilience skills and strategies, as well as many ways to practice and then to incorporate them into daily life. (Some are listed in Chapter 2, but see Reivich and Shatté, 2002, for a fuller list.) These skills are closely related and interdependent, with powerful mutual influences. The following four skills probably are most immediately accessible to parents and families:[3]

- Learning the importance of taking risks
- Recognizing and regulating emotions—comprising two components: learning to identify feelings and then learning to control one's emotional responses to events and situations
- Learning to trust oneself, to count on one's strengths, and to develop a sense of mastery
- Learning the importance of reaching out to others

Each of these skills is discussed briefly next.

### *Risk Taking*

For many people, simply attending a workshop amounts to taking a risk. Thus, no special exercise is suggested, and in its place, the concept of taking risks and its importance in living with disabilities serves as the first discussion topic. (It is certainly possible, however, to devise such an exercise if the group leader wishes to do

---

[3]You may wish to choose others, but the point is to provide exercises that you believe illustrate simple resilience techniques that can be profitably applied to and by parents of communicatively disordered children.

so.) The facilitator may begin the session by noting that the participants were not ordered to come to these sessions, nor were any promises made about the workshop's outcome—yet here they are, in what (before the last session at least) was a step, if not a full-fledged leap, into an unknown experience. Some potential questions for the discussion include the following:

- Why did you come?
- What are your expectations?
- What risks did you take just to be here?
- How does stepping off into the unknown relate to having children with disabilities? To living with adults who have them?
- Is taking risks a necessity?
- What risks have you taken? In general? In relation to your child or family member?
- What does risk-taking have to do with resilience?

A discussion of questions such as these leads directly into some exercises designed to illustrate resilience and to practice some of its skills.

### Activity One: Recognizing and Regulating Emotions

The "Recognizing and Regulating Emotions" exercise is designed to help participants gain control of emotional responses in stressful personal interactions and events. Every life has stressors and stresses, but ample evidence indicates that they are disproportionate for parents and families living with disability. There are many ways to deal with stress, but common to most of them are calming techniques, ranging from taking a few deep breaths, to learning to manage breathing, to systematic progressive relaxation. These *stepping back* approaches permit the person experiencing stress to take stock of the situation and attempt to put it into perspective. This workshop provides practice for a simple and quite effective approach, similar to the pauses discussed in Chapter 3 as important for communication counselors to learn to use before replying to clients.

Workshop participants are taught a set of specific techniques to use in handling a negative stressful event: (1) Immediately identify and name the feeling—that is, identify the initial emotional response.[4] (2) Then, before responding, take a deep breath, instruct yourself to calm down, and wait for 20 seconds. During that time, think of alternative responses—it does not matter, at this point, whether these alternative responses are positive or negative. (3) Then reevaluate the initial reaction, and perhaps modify it before responding by word or action.

■ This takes practice, but fortunately all the practice does not have to be on the firing line, as it were. All of us have experienced stressful situations when we wish we had reacted differently, and one form of practice is to mentally replay some of those old instances and imagine a different response. It also can be instructive to read advice columns in the newspaper. Because the content of the letters and responses typically is emotionally charged, an interesting exercise is to register one's emotions and responses while reading the column and then compare them with the recommendations of "Dear Abby" or another columnist. Another approach is to practice with scenarios. Box 8.4 contains four examples: two for parents and two for families.

### *Activity Two:* Learning to Trust Yourself

*Self-efficacy* is the fancy word for trusting yourself, knowing your strengths and how you can use them to cope with adversity and to solve problems. Few people believe they can handle every task, although most are pretty sure of their ability to come through in some. The hard ones are the tough situations, but if they look at

---

[4]You may wish to begin this exercise by simply having the group provide names for a variety of negative emotions, such as fear, anger, guilt, jealousy, or disappointment. You can work this activity up and down the age scale, incidentally—for example, by asking children to name emotions, and then recognize them from various film clips, and so on.

### Box 8.4 Week 2: Recognizing and Regulating Emotions Exercise

The group leader reads a scenario and asks participants to write down their emotional responses, immediately, before thinking about it. Then the leader asks participants to think about their responses and come up with some alternatives. Each scenario is discussed in turn, with volunteers from the group contributing their suggestions. Relevant questions may include the following:

- Why is it important to recognize and control emotional responses?

Once you have practiced it for a while, how can you pass this skill on to other members of the family (including your children)?

**Parent Version**

1. Your 9-year-old daughter was crying when she got off the school bus. She reported that three other girls from the neighborhood had teased her "all the way home" because she came from the special class. They also told her, she says, that she was "funny looking."
2. You and your wife have been researching cochlear implants for your 6-month-old son Victor, who has a severe hearing impairment According to some of the extensive material you have read, implementation can occur as early as 12 months. You both are eager to have the surgery as soon as possible. You schedule a visit to the cochlear implant clinic in the medical center closest to your home, where Victor is evaluated. Both the pediatric otolaryngologist and the audiologist tell you that they cannot be sure at this point that Victor is a candidate, and that in any event, they will not consider implementation until he is reevaluated at age 2.

**Family Version**

1. Your aphasic family member's most vexing problem since his stroke is that he has not been permitted to drive again.

You are not very happy about it either, because you must do all the driving. Your physician finally gives you permission to seek out a retraining program for handicapped drivers. You schedule an appointment with the driving training person, and when you arrive, she tells you that she does not train people with language problems because she does not believe that they can be counted on to drive safely.

2. You and your spouse have always been part of a traditional family Thanksgiving dinner that rotates from home to home in your extensive family. Your sister, who is this year's hostess, tells you that it would be "better for all" if you did not bring your wife, who has moderate AD, to this year's dinner, "because it makes everyone so sad to see her that way."

self-mastery overall, people are likely to see their character strengths shining through. My own experience furnishes an illustration:

I happen to have Angel Food Cake Self-Efficacy (AFCSE). With the level of competence I have managed to attain, I trust myself to produce a perfect cake every time. A look back on how I achieved AFCSE showed a combination of contributing factors: (1) It took practice; (2) it happened in small steps, not all at once; and (3) it was notably enhanced by using my signature strengths—humor, curiosity, and love of learning. So what if I bombed early on? Even Julia Child acknowledged that it took her practice to learn a lot of things.

Cake #1 was a disaster, but I knew enough to laugh about it, and I wanted to improve. At Cake #2, curiosity and love of learning kicked in: How will I know when the egg whites are just right? How do I know a flat cake tastes bad? By Cake #3, I was onto the "folding process" (again, curiosity, love of learning, and I was still chuckling over my improving but less-than-perfect product). By #5, I was home free: perfection. I had achieved AFCSE. And not only that, AFCSE generalized to lemon soufflés.

Self-efficacy is an important ingredient of resilience, as well as an essential quality in developing into an authoritative (not authoritarian) parent for one's children. Like many other personal qualities and skills, it is particularly useful in parenting children at risk for disabilities and in living with family members who have incurred disabilities. Not only is self-efficacy developed in small steps, but it probably starts in self-recognition of mastery of a few simple small things, like baking an angel food cake. Box 8.5 is a useful exercise for kick-starting self-efficacy and mastery.

After group members complete the exercise, discussion can focus on the following points.

■ For parents, are there some important implications for role modeling self-trust for the family?

---

**Box 8.5 Week 2: Trusting Yourself Exercise— Parent and Family Version**

Each of us recognizes our mastery of something, however small. This *self-efficacy* serves to put us on the path to trust ourselves to handle bigger ones. Describe one thing you can count on yourself to do well. How did you apply the three principles of practice, small steps, and applying one or more of your strengths?

**Parent Version**

Think of some aspect of your child-raising to which you could apply these principles. Find a way to use the steps to teach your child a task that he or she can perform with confidence.

**Family Version**

Think of a small task, not necessarily communication related, that your spouse may be able to do successfully (or reassume the responsibility for) (e.g., separating coins by size and putting them in a coin dispenser, feeding the fish, balancing the checkbook). Help him or her to follow the three principles of practice, small steps, and applying a strength to do or resume doing the task.

---

■ Is it likely that your children will also benefit from developing self-trust? How can you help them to develop it?

■ For families, how might your self-efficacy improve the situation for your disabled partner?

■ How might you help your spouse to gain or regain some mastery?

### *Activity Three:* Reaching Out

Resilience is not a matter of taking what comes one's way, toughing it out, being the master of one's fate. This attribute is defined at some length in Chapter 2, but it also can be thought of simply as the "capacity to maintain competent function in the face of major life stressors" (Masten, Best, & Garmezy, 1990). Resilience involves many skills, as suggested previously, and reaching out is a critical one, both to check on one's perceptions and to position oneself to receive help from others. Reaching out, of course, also involves being able to accept the reaching out of others, of learning to be honored and empowered by it. Box 8.6 contains an exercise that is designed as a first step to reaching out.

This is the final exercise for this session. Typically, everyone finds someone to reach out to, but the group leader may need to broker this process, either by getting some of the "strays" together or by personally reaching out to anyone who has not yet made contact with another participant. The exercise should take no more than

---

#### Box 8.6 Week 2: Reaching Out Exercise

By now, you probably have noticed one person (at least) in the workshop whose comments have moved or impressed you, and whom you would like to get to know a little better. Or perhaps you have been touched by someone's problems and wish to find out more, if only to help a bit. Or perhaps you have been concerned about a person in the room who has been very shy and has difficulty speaking. Now reach out to that person in keeping with the basis for your interest—explore or share an insight, give a hug or a pat on the back, or encourage with supportive words.

10 or so minutes. This is a "feel good" interaction for everyone, and one that provides an easy transition to discussion. Appropriate discussion questions include the following:

- Is there a balance between reaching out and going it alone?
- Can reaching out be giving as well as seeking?
- Reaching out also means finding support groups and websites. Does anyone have some they particularly wish to share? (The group leader may wish to make available as a handout a list of some of the websites from previous chapters that may be helpful.)

### Homework: Three Good Things Exercise

Box 8.7 presents another version of the Three Good Things exercise described in Chapter 2. It is particularly appropriate here because it combines aspects of self-efficacy, in understanding the role an individual plays in causing positive emotions; reaching out, in version by recognizing others' roles. As before, the leader's role is to explain the exercise, and encourage participants to write up their experiences, in terms of what they have learned from it.

## Week 3

The major focus of Week 3 is on how to develop "optimistic explanatory style" (Peterson, 2006; Peterson & Steen, 2005; Reivich & Shatté, 2002), part of the fabric of positive psychology. Explanatory style in its essence involves the perceptions and understandings people use in explaining events to themselves, how those explanations influence their behavior, and how they can, with practice, learn to recognize and change them, and as a result think more optimistically. The exercises that preceded Week 3 all have contributed to the process of improved self-awareness. But because explanatory style is not particularly transparent, but often hidden deep in personal belief systems and characteristic responses, this component of positive psychology is addressed directly here, along with finding some ways to challenge underlying beliefs. Communication counselors

---

### Box 8.7 Week 2: Homework—Three Good Things

**Parent Version**

- Begin each day this week by selecting a member of your family (spouse, child, yourself). Find a way to keep track, either by observation or asking, of three good things that happened to the chosen person each day. What did the person do to bring them about?
- Share this information with the chosen person at the end of the day.

**Family Version**

- For three days this week, focus on your disabled family member. Either by observing or asking, find three good things that happened to him or her on those days. Before you go to bed, share your thoughts on what he or she did to bring them about.
- For three other days, focus on yourself. At the end of the day, summarize them to yourself, and determine what you did to bring them about.
- For the final day, turn the tables. Observe one good thing that happened to you today that came about because of something your family member did. Also, observe one good thing that happened to him or her because of something *you* did. Share the information before going to bed.

---

are urged to revisit Chapter 2 but also to explore Reivich and Shatté (2002) once again, to broaden their understanding of explanatory style beyond the simple introduction provided here.

Week 3 begins with a short lecture, highlighting the following main points: When bad things happen to people, particularly events out of their control, they frequently experience feelings of helplessness. Having a child with a handicap can be such a situation, and as parents struggle to understand and to move with it, they attempt to understand why it has happened. This also is the situation for families when a family member experiences a catastrophic medical event. These are major adversities, but in daily life, many smaller but nevertheless upsetting adversities occur as well.

What each person brings to adversity (major or minor) is explanatory style—how that person explains adversity to himself or herself. Explanatory style tends to emerge from three sources: (1) internal factors versus external factors; (2) factors of permanence versus change; and (3) global factors versus local factors. Reivich and Shatté summarize these three factors colloquially as "me versus not me," "always versus sometimes," and "everything versus not everything," respectively. Each is briefly described next.

*Me versus not me* sets the locus of responsibility: "I am totally responsible for all that happens—good and bad—not only to me but also to those around me, and possibly in extreme cases, for everything that happens in my world." People with this outlook see themselves as those who bring these events about. For example, a "me" person may state: "It is my fault that Gustav had his stroke, because I didn't insist that he take it easy. He was working too hard, and I knew it." Conversely, a "not me" person takes little responsibility for what happens to him or her or their immediate others. It is the fault of someone or something else.

*Always versus seldom* sets the temporal locus. For example, someone at the extremes sees all events as unique at one pole or the way things always are—good and bad—at the other. Use of the words "never" and "always" is a good indicator of this style. Statements such as "Nothing like this illness has ever happened before to us" and "Illness and pain have always been a part of my experience" also provide some clues to this explanatory style.

Finally there is the durability, or generalization, of *everything versus not everything*—the notion of "the way it always is" versus "unique to this one event." "This is the story of my life" implies "everything." "Nothing in my life prepared me for this" implies "not everything."

All three factors are end points on a range; few people are at the extremes. In adversity-laden situations, however, people who are "addicted" to pessimism crowd around the *me, always, everything* end of the range, whereas cockeyed optimists are at the other end.

The first exercise related to these continua appears as Box 8.8. The goal is to help workshop participants situate themselves along each of the three continua, and to discuss how these reactions fuel their beliefs. Provide paper and use the examples in Box 8.8 to have participants rate themselves on the three dimensions.

### Box 8.8 Week 3: "Me-Always-Everything" Examples

**Parent Version**

*Example 1*

At the insistence of your family and your pediatrician, you made an appointment to have your child evaluated by the city's leading neuropsychologist. It took 6 months to get the appointment, and today is the big day, but your child woke up with a temperature of 103 degrees, and you have to cancel the appointment. How could this have happened?

*Belief*: I should have been very careful to keep him out of drafts and away from kids who were not well, so that he would have been shipshape today.

Is this a good explanation for you? Rate it on the following scale:

**Totally due to me**                    **Just circumstance**

| 1 | 2 | 3 | 4 | 5 | 6 | 7 |

*Belief*: It's probably silly to make another appointment, because it will just happen again.

**Such stuff always happens**    **It won't happen again**

| 1 | 2 | 3 | 4 | 5 | 6 | 7 |

*Belief*: That's the way life is. I can't win.

**It's the story of my life**    **A unique circumstance**

| 1 | 2 | 3 | 4 | 5 | 6 | 7 |

*Example 2*

You had a really hard day at work, and when you got home, you discovered that your 10-year-old had misplaced her house key, so she went to the neighbor's, where she watched TV instead of doing her homework. She also couldn't do her chore for the day, which was to take dinner out of the freezer, and you have no backup supper dish. You threw a fit.

*Belief*: **I expect too much from my kids**                    **It was all her fault**

| 1 | 2 | 3 | 4 | 5 | 6 | 7 |

*Belief*: **That's the**
**way it's gonna be**

| | | | | | It will never happen again |
|---|---|---|---|---|---|

    1    2    3    4    5    6    7

*Belief*: **Everything**
**goes this way**                     **It's a unique event**

    1    2    3    4    5    6    7

**Family Version**

*Example 1*

Since Hugh's stroke, you have had to go back to work, and be responsible for getting him to therapy, being sure he's picked up by the Handi-Car service at the right time, and brought home again every day. You ask your sister to check in to see that all is going off on schedule. You come home on Wednesday after a hard day, and Hugh is not there. The new Handi-Car driver forgot to pick him up and the speech clinic secretary calls to ask when you are going to pick him up.

*Belief*: **This is my fault—**
**I should have reminded my**         **My sister is**
**sister to remind the driver**        **a ditz brain**

    1    2    3    4    5    6    7

*Belief*: **It's always**              **All will be well**
**this way—nothing**       **when the new driver**
**goes right**                 **learns the ropes**

    1    2    3    4    5    6    7

*Belief*: **This stroke is**          **Some snafus are**
**ruining our whole life**        **bound to occur**

    1    2    3    4    5    6    7

*Example 2*

Your neighbor calls to tell you that your wife, Alice, who has mild dementia, is walking alone down the street in her nightgown, asking everyone the way to the church you both used to attend, and that it's Sunday and she is late for services (it's Wednesday).

*Belief:* **It's all my fault—
how did I not notice
she'd left?**

**Not my fault—
she must have found
the front door key**

1    2    3    4    5    6    7

*Belief:* **I've gotta keep an
eye on her all the time**

**A new lock will
take care of it**

1    2    3    4    5    6    7

*Belief:* **Soon she
will be wandering
everywhere**

**Church was so
important to her—this
was an isolated event**

1    2    3    4    5    6    7

After the rating has been completed, the discussion should focus on points such as the following:

- How beliefs influence behavior. Use the example situations as stimuli for generating alternative actions. Refer back to Box 8.4, which presents an exercise on recognizing feelings.
- How we can generate alternatives to them, again referring back to the feelings exercise.
- The danger of extremes at each end of the continuum.

An important implication of this kind of analysis is how we explain the relationship between adversities, beliefs and consequences, and how we can learn to change our behavior in relation to them. (A), ourselves stands for the adversities, (B) represents our beliefs in relationship to them and (C) stands for the negative emotional consequences of those beliefs. Reivich and Shatté (2002) lay out a potent grid for examining the consequences of adversity, modulated by beliefs:

| **The Belief** | **Its Consequences** |
|---|---|
| Violation of one's rights | Anger |
| Real-world loss, or loss of self-worth | Sadness, depression |
| Violation of another's rights | Guilt |

| The Belief | Its Consequences |
| --- | --- |
| Future threat | Anxiety |
| Negative self-comparison with others | Embarrassment |

To learn to change one's responses to adversity, whether for parents dealing with the teacher who doesn't quite understand their concerns about their child or for a family member dealing with a doctor who cannot predict a time course for recovery from TBI, one has first to understand these connections. The next step is examining the connections, and to provide oneself with counter-arguments (disputing them is the D component of this approach) that encourage flexibility in problem solving and developing resilience. This is the ABCD of "hot seating" (Peterson, 2006) or of developing "real-time resilience" (Reivich & Shatté, 2002).

## Developing Alternative Ways of Thinking: The ABCD Approach

The second exercise, and a pivotal one, begins the process of confronting one's explanatory style. Essentially, the approach involves learning to (1) evaluate the evidence for one's immediate response; (2) think of alternative ways of explaining the situation; and (3) use these alternatives as the basis for developing a different approach to the adversity. The crucial questions are as follows:

- What alternatives are available as explanations?
- Can I practice arguing with my initial reaction? Can I come up with alternative explanations?
- What difference would it make? Is there value in changing my response?
- How can I apply this to my life?

Peterson (2006) suggests using another trusted person, aware of the process, to provide counterpoint and aid in developing alternatives. Although practicing with another may be necessary for some persons early on, once they have identified their own explanatory style, and have practiced often enough, most people can (and in the long run should) serve this function for themselves.[5]

Box 8.9 presents two extended examples, one for parents of a moderately handicapped child with cerebral palsy and one for family members—in this case the spouse of an aphasic man. These examples provide problem-oriented material for discussion in their respective workshops. A useful follow-up exercise is to have workshop participants pair off and continue practice, as described in Box 8.10.

The session ends with an exercise based on the gratitude visit, one of the most moving of the exercises for which Seligman, Steen, Park, and Peterson (2005) have provided efficacy data. This exercise, introduced in Chapter 2, is simply the act of remembering someone to whom you are especially grateful, and whom you have never properly thanked for whatever this person has done for you. Once you have chosen your recipient, write a short (i.e., one page or so) letter of gratitude; then schedule a meeting or a phone call and simply read the letter aloud to the person being thanked. Then evaluate the effects not only on the person but also on yourself.

The gratitude visit becomes the first assignment of the week— that is, to plan and carry out a gratitude visit. The second is to apply "real-time resilience" in a few instances that arise during the week. Both of these assignments should be recorded in the notebook or on evaluation sheets.

---

### Box 8.9  Week 3 Problem-Oriented Issues for Illustrating ABCD: Family and Parent Version

***Example 1*** "Real-Time Resilience": Adults
The following resilience approach for aphasic adults is based on Reivich and Shatté's ABCD approach (2002).

---

[5]From a personal perspective, I have learned and I practice "real-time resilience" or perhaps (apologies to Peterson) "personal hot seating." Although it took a lot of careful practice early on, I can attest that it became easier and is now almost automatic almost two years later. One of its joys is that mental "hot seating" is serviceable for concerns as diverse as why I have had an unsatisfactory interaction with a coaching client and as why my garbage disposal once again is giving me fits.

**The problem:** "I can't leave him alone. What if he had another stroke?"

**The goal:** Dissect into adversity (A), beliefs (B), consequences (C); then dispute them (D).

### The View of Spouse Jennifer

A = ADVERSITY: George had a stroke and can't talk.

B = BELIEF: I can't leave him alone, because what if he had another stroke?

*Uncovered thinking trap* and connection between beliefs and consequences:

If he has another stroke, and I'm not there to get help, I am afraid he will die. I will be responsible for his death.

C = CONSEQUENCES

*Emotional consequences*:

I feel anxious. I will be responsible for his death.

I am angry. I have to take George everywhere I go.

*Behavioral consequences*:

That's no fun for either of us.

I am trapped.

I don't have any time to myself.

D = DISPUTATION: Let's think this through.

- Is this realistic? What are the odds?
- Does George have any safeguards in place in case he needs help? (e.g., augmentative devices, medical alert system, panic button on house alarm). The answer is yes—all of these.
- Does Jennifer have any back-up alternatives? Friends, children, help in house who could give her free time? The answer is yes.
- Does Jennifer know how George views this state of affairs? The answer is no.

### The View of George, the Severely Aphasic Spouse

A = ADVERSITY: Jennifer won't leave me alone since the stroke.

B = BELIEF: She thinks I'm incompetent.

*Uncovered thinking trap*: If my wife of 30 years thinks I'm incompetent, I must be.

C = CONSEQUENCES

*Emotional consequences*:

I am angry with Jennifer for not believing in me.

I am frustrated because I have no choices.

I am sad because I am incompetent.

*Behavioral consequences*:

I have to go everywhere that Jennifer goes.

I feel trapped.

I don't have any time to myself.

D = DISPUTATION

Because George is severely aphasic, probably the foregoing intact internal dialogue cannot be expressed, or will be expressed in emotional ways (registering anger, frustration, and sadness). Therefore, the disputation is largely in Jennifer's terms. Each of her points can be disputed, as follows: Does George's anger and frustration make sense? Yes, it does. Jennifer's behavior belies his cognitive competence. Another stroke is possible, certainly, but regular doctor visits are in place, medications are taken systematically, and he does not need constant supervision during speech therapy. And nobody checks on his opinion.

- Is George incompetent? No, he just can't talk.
- Are there safeguards? George has a backup, simple augmentative system for calling 911 and also has a medical alert system in place.
- Family and friends have offered to stay with George but have never been called on.
- Because it is not easy to get George's side, a clinician may play George's part, as described. George ideally is present for this and is encouraged to agree or disagree.

Develop a plan of action in three steps:

1. Validate George's point of view.
2. Use appropriate questions, or have a clinician role-play George's part, as described previously. George is present and encouraged to agree or disagree.

3. Test the realities uncovered in the disputation.
   - Call in the daughter-in-law to stay with George while Jennifer goes to the beauty shop. Did George have a stroke? Repeat as necessary to collect data. Then try successive trips away alone (e.g., take a 5-minute walk, go to the Starbuck's on the corner and bring George a cup of his favorite coffee, go for a 15-minute walk) Collect the data. Evaluate everyone's feelings.
   - Help Jennifer to learn the technique so that she can do it on her own for other situations. You may wish to use the technique yourself to address one of your own problems—experience using it helps you to explain it.

*Example 2* "Real-Time Resilience": Children
The following resilience approach developed for the parents of Halston, a 6-year-old boy with moderate-severe cerebral palsy including dysarthria, is based on Reivich and Shatté's ABCD approach (2002).

> **The problem:** The school wants to mainstream Halston for first grade.
> **The goal:** Dissect into adversity (A), beliefs (B), consequences (C); then dispute them (D).

**The View of Parents Ada and Clark**

A = ADVERSITY: His schoolmates will not accept Halston.

B = BELIEFS:

Halston needs to be protected.

He doesn't understand.

We, not the school, should be making this decision.

*Uncovered thinking traps* and connections between beliefs and consequences:

We have invested great energy in making his world safe. This investment will be lost.

Down underneath it all, we have doubts about Halston's abilities.

Our rights are being violated.

C = CONSEQUENCES

*Emotional consequences*:
We feel anxious.
We feel angry.
We are embarrassed.

*Behavioral consequences*:
We are confronting the school.

D = DISPUTATION: Let's think this through.

- Is this realistic? What are the odds?
- The school has tested Halston. They feel he is fine.
- Has Halston been okay in his interactions with other children? The answer is yes.
- Are there other things as important as being protected? The answer is yes—such things include acceptance by others, which can't happen without trying.
- Is there help available for Halston and us? Yes.

Develop a plan of action with two steps:

1. Test the realities uncovered in the disputation.
   - Before school starts, invite some of his potential classmates over to play. See what happens. Get the data.
   - Check with your older children.
   - Talk to the school about your concerns; gain assurance of their help. Develop an acceptable alterative plan together with the school.
   - Find out what Halston thinks about going to first grade.
2. Help Ada and Clark learn the technique so that they can use it in other situations. You may wish to use the technique yourself to address one of your own problems—experience using it helps you to explain it.

*Note*: This adversity has been less fully described than that involving George and Jennifer, primarily because the model is transparent enough to permit easy elaboration. Notice that this one has many possible permutations. For example, what if Ada and Clark differed in their opinions about whether or not to mainstream Halston? And what about Halston's own opinions? those of his siblings?

> ### Box 8.10 Week 3: Pair-off Practice with "Real-Time Resilience"
>
> Any of the scenarios described in Box 8.4 or Box 8.8 can serve as adversity examples (or, for that matter, many of the "counseling moments"). This pairing-off exercise concerns what beliefs are triggered by the adversity and the consequences that follow. One participant takes the role of the person who has had the adversity; the other, the role of the colleague who helps figure out alternatives to the beliefs. When the necessary goals have been achieved for the selected adversity example, the participants switch roles. It also is possible, even preferable, for people to describe and to work through their own adversities. Group leaders are encouraged to be as creative as possible in developing scenarios. By now, the workshop participants have become pretty well known to each other, and appropriate scenarios can be developed for specific pairings of participants.

## Week 4: Wrap-up

Week 4 is intended to be an uplifting and very pleasant informal experience. The goal is to launch participants into further explorations in the arena of living as fully and authentically as possible, and supporting their continued use of the kinds of resilience-building activities that are the focus of the workshop. The first activity of the week, then, is to share the experiences the group has had in planning and carrying out their gratitude visits. This usually is a momentous and significant activity for most members of the group, who seem at first surprised to find that they have gotten perhaps even more than they have given as they planned and carried out the exercise. Discussion points are many and varied and include at least the following:

- Can you consider making other gratitude visits? For example, is there someone who has been particularly helpful to you in dealing with your child or your spouse? What about thanking some members of your own family?

■ Gratitude visits often are costly in terms of planning and execution. What are other, simpler ways to similar (if less dramatic) ends?

■ Why is expressing gratitude so powerful?

Experiences in changing explanatory style through real-time resilience and hot seating also should be examined. These experiences can initiate a general discussion of what individuals have learned or achieved from the workshop, and how future workshops can be improved. The facilitator may wish to provide handouts that will help people continue to apply what they have learned in the workshop. Many additional exercises can be found throughout this book. The suggestions inspired by Masten and Reed (2005), and presented in Box 8.11, can be used as an effective handout for parents.

It is important at the last session to leave enough time for interpersonal networking and visiting, and it is my preference is to

---

### Box 8.11 Week 4: Strategies for Promoting Resilience in Children with Disabilities*

■ Build self-efficacy through small steps; practice simple things first.
■ Teach coping strategies for specific situations.
■ Foster secure attachment relationships between you and your child.
■ Seek help from other families and other experts.
■ Participate in programs designed for special needs children in your community
■ Seek trustworthy support from Internet resources.
■ Help your child to establish friendships with other children.
■ Support cultural traditions that provide children with adaptive rituals and opportunities to bond with other children and adults (e.g., religious education, Little League, Special Olympics).

*Inspired by Masten and Reed (2005).

conclude with refreshments and enough time to tie up loose ends informally. Workshops invariably provide an intense learning experience for both facilitators and participants. Therefore, the group leader may wish to conclude with his or her own gratitude statement to the participants.

# VARIATIONS ON THE WORKSHOP THEME

## Adolescents Who Stutter

The format for this workshop variant remains the same. The exercises, from the parents and family versions, can easily be adapted for use with adolescents who stutter or, for that matter, with adolescents with TBI. In addition to these, the exercises that concluded Chapter 5 almost without exception can be fitted into the framework of this workshop. For example, exercises number 8, 9, and 10, are all versions of the gratitude visit; the mishap scenarios from the laugh lesson exercise can be used for real time resilience; exercises number 4 and 7 both fit well into the theme of building trust in oneself. Possibly the biggest difference from the more standard format is that communication counselors should be especially alert to fostering strong peer relationships among participants throughout the workshop. Because these focused workshops are likely to be small, this should not be difficult. It also usually is possible to pay closer attention to individual participants' needs. Because, as previously discussed, there is some emerging evidence of the effectiveness of cognitive-behavioral therapy (CBT) in the management of stuttering, one goal of this workshop, in addition to the general goals discussed previously, may be to encourage some group members to participate in CBT.

## Adults with Aphasia

Again, the explicit format of the workshop experience for adults with aphasia should not differ markedly in terms either the topics covered or the types of exercises undertaken. The family variant, rather than the parent variant, is used. Once again, counselors are encouraged to revisit previous chapters for appropriate exercises that have been especially adapted for persons with aphasia.

Although the format may not vary significantly, implementation for adults with aphasia will require some modifications. First, it probably is not possible to do all of the exercises and discuss them fully in the constrained time frame, unless participation is limited to persons with mild aphasia. Because people with more moderate problems, and even some with severe aphasias, can profit from this experience, one solution is to use fewer exercises.

Another variation may be to double the number of sessions, but it seems more appropriate simply to repeat the experience for those who are interested, and change the exercises in the second series. Another recommended modification is to limit group size to 10 to 12 participants, to ensure balanced participation. Finally, this workshop variation must include "supported communication" procedures, and to ensure implementation of this support, at least two group leaders are necessary.

## Conclusions

In writing this chapter, I continually had to remind myself that I was preparing not an experimental protocol or a series of lesson plans but rather a set of definitive guidelines for creating meaningful workshop experiences for adults and children who have communication disorders, and for their significant others. Nevertheless, clinicians interested in conducting such a workshop are urged to collect as much information as possible concerning its utility. Both qualitative and quantitative data are appropriate. Workshops such as these are perhaps the most significant departures from traditional approaches to the management of speech, language, and hearing disorders that have been discussed in this book, yet they have potential for increasing the quality of life for the clients we serve. If they are to be viable, supporting documentation is mandatory.

## References

Masten, A. S., & Reed, M.-G. (2005). Resilience in development. In C. Snyder & S. Lopez (Eds.), *Handbook of positive psychology.* Oxford: Oxford University Press.

Masten, A. S., Best, K. M., & Garmezy, N. (1990). Resilience and development: Contributions from the study of children who overcome adversity. *Development and Psychopathology, 2,* 425–244.

Peterson, C. (2006). *A primer in positive psychology.* New York: Oxford University Press.

Reivich, K., & Shatté, A. (2002). *The resilience factor: Seven essential skills for overcoming life's inevitable obstacles.* New York: Broadway Books.

Seligman, M. (2002). *Authentic happiness.* New York: Free Press.

Seligman, M. E. P., Steen, T. A., Park, N., & Peterson, C. (2005). Positive psychology progress: Empirical validation of interventions. *American Psychologist, 60*(5), 410–421.

## Chapter 9

# THERE'S AN ELEPHANT IN THE ROOM: ISSUES IN DEATH AND DYING

## Stan Goldberg, PhD

## Foreword

It seems totally fitting that this book on counseling across the lifespan should conclude with a chapter on end-of-life issues dealt with positively and directly. Today's clinicians who work in extended care facilities increasingly encounter clients who are dying, but little in their coursework has prepared them for the experience of the death of a person with whom they have formed a rather intimate association. In my own counseling courses, I have relied on Stan Goldberg, who once was my student and now is my teacher in this and many other topics, to guide me. His experiences as a hospice worker and as a gifted communication counselor and clinician make him a uniquely qualified authority on the issues of death and dying in communication counseling. Initially I had asked him only for help with this chapter; when later he graciously volunteered to write it himself, I accepted it as the gift of loving-kindness that it is. Read it with care and respect.

ALH

## Introduction

Death is like the strange relative we speak about in whispers, and then only when children aren't present. Even though we try to keep it from conscious thought, discomfort bubbles up when we encounter a patient who is obviously dying. We tell her how good she looks, despite her sunken cheeks and sallow complexion. We're tongue-tied—not because we don't care, but because we fear death.

Those who are courageous enough to hold the gaze may read books such as Elisabeth Kübler-Ross's *On Death and Dying* (Kübler-Ross, 1997). In it and others equally insightful, the process of dying is calmly and objectively explained. But as the linguist Korzybski said, "The map is not the territory" (Korzybski, 1958). Death can't be known through dispassionate reading. Nor is it grasped by discussing "management" issues such as hospital rules, universal precautions, Medicare billing policies, demographics, or practices based on the American Speech-Language-Hearing Association's (ASHA) code of ethics. No, the experience of death is personal—an event so rich, that just like a gourmet dish, it cannot be adequately described through words. I won't try to do it in this chapter. Instead, the chapter explores events and emotional states that surround death, and how you can have a significant impact on the quality of your patient's life, whether it is measured in months or even hours.

There is a Tibetan saying that to get over those things that are feared the most, draw them in close (Patrul Rinpoche, 1994). And how to get chummy with death is the theme of this chapter, which looks at what communication counselors can contribute to dying patients, and what you, as a human being, can learn from the experience.

## Why Practice Speech or Language Therapy with the Dying?

I remember a conversation I had with my mother when I decided to become a speech-language pathologist (SLP). She was a wonderful but simple woman. As she got older, there were things she had difficulty understanding—like my choice of profession. "Speech-language pathology?" she asked. "What's that?" After carefully explaining what I did, I thought she understood until I heard her talking to a friend: "He's a speech-language pathologist. You know, someone who helps children move their tongues." No, she didn't get it right 30-some years ago. But as I look at ASHA's current scope of practice for SLPs, I find her description prophetic. We have moved in the direction of being highly competent specialists—technically more precise, but now maybe less willing to go beyond moving tongues (Goldberg, 2003).

## Scope of Practice

We've strayed from the first visions our professions' founders had more than 70 years ago. Although they wanted us to correct speech and language problems, they also believed we had another obligation to our clients. They viewed the people they served as whole human beings, who needed not only technical services but also compassion. (Therapy for the dying is not about technical competency—*it's about facilitating painful communications.*

When people near their own death, suppressed emotions and fears surface as if the barriers confining them became porous. As a hospice volunteer, I was with a woman in her 90s who vividly remembered the beatings her mother gave her when she was 5 years of age. She repeated the story to each person caring for her in a hospice facility, even acting it out when morphine made her delirious. Although I was there as a bedside volunteer, my training and experience as a speech-language pathologist enabled me to help her communicate her pain, not only to others but also to herself.

## Competency in Communication

As professionals, we have become prisoners of our name. Years ago, we were "speech pathologists." As the importance of differentiating between language and speech problems gained momentum, we became "speech-language pathologists." Now, we call ourselves "aphasiologists," or "early language interventionists," or "speech-language pathologists with an emphasis in _____" (fill in the blank). The increasing narrowing of how we identify ourselves reflects a changing focus on what we do, or are willing to do.

We focus on correcting specific speech and language disorders as if that were the final goal—but it's not. Speech and language are just *tools* of communication. We work on helping our clients develop and use these tools to facilitate communication. When we dwell less on our newly acquired parochialism, our competency in correcting specific disorders becomes the means for achieving a greater goal. We become *communication counselors*, who also are competent to work on helping clients develop and use their tools for communicating.

## Painful Communications: What Are They?

A number of years ago at a workshop, Sogyal Rinpoche (1993) related a conversation a counselor had with a dying patient. The patient said he didn't need to have anyone understand what he was going through; that wasn't possible. Rather, he just wanted people to *act* as if they did. I don't claim special knowledge when it comes to death, although I've taken the journey often with others. Like everyone else, I'll need to wait until it's my turn to really know what it's about. But as a hospice volunteer, I've seen reoccurring communication problems emanating from the impending experience of death in both children and adults. It's possible to do more than just act as if we understand what our patient is experiencing.

The initial step is understanding that the dying process is messy, both physically and psychologically. By its very nature, it continually changes, moving persons through the most dramatic changes they will experience (Goldberg, 2006). Change is difficult for most people to accept, even under ordinary circumstances. When change occurs gradually, it can be made more acceptable (Goldberg, 1997). But with terminal illnesses, change occurs as if it sits on an out-of-control conveyer belt, ignoring the wishes of the person whose life it is changing.

With lingering terminal illnesses, personalities change by necessity—rarely by choice. As people are forced to move from independence to dependence, health to illness, being in control to having none, their world becomes contorted, as does their place in it. The difficulties they encounter often become apparent when they try to communicate their psychological pain. Four recurring themes are adjusting to changes, expressing gratitude, regrets, and the need to simplify. Within each of these areas of concern, communication counselors have the power to alleviate suffering.

## Unsettling Nature of Change

For the person who is dying, a world that may have been as solid as concrete becomes as unstable as a bowl of Jell-O. Tibetans have a word for this rootless psychological state. They call it the *bardo* (Sogyal Rinpoche, 1994). Although the term is traditionally reserved for the time between death and the consciousness leaving the body, it can be applied to transitions from who a person was to who that person is becoming (Goldberg, 2002). There is discomfort in transitions, sometimes even fear. People are moving from something they know to an unknown. Some people believe the fear of death may have more to do with giving up what's familiar than with dreading the last breath and what happens afterward (Krishnamurti, 1994).

I've witnessed family members and friends unable to understand such changes. Knowing the person was dying, they still expected that person to act the same as before getting sick. When the kind, happy, accepting person becomes belligerent and is no longer interested in anything but his or her own memories, support from puzzled family members often vanishes. Communication counselors can enable the person who is dying to express the fears he or she may be feeling. And if they can't, your obligation is to convey this fact to family and friends.

### *What to Do*

- Expect your patients to have sudden mood shifts.
- Don't minimize the changes they are experiencing.
- If patients ask what it's like to die, tell them—if you know. If you do not, find someone who has been with people who have died.
- Don't initiate discussions about dying. When patients are ready to talk about it, they'll let you know.
- Accept every change in your patient's personality. Don't expect consistency.

- Help patients express the fear they are experiencing to friends and family.
- When patients can't express their fear, you should convey it to family and friends.

## Gratitude—Giving and Receiving

Accepting gratitude can be a public statement of personal need. The grateful person who is dying may be saying "I can't do it anymore by myself." For people who have taken pride in being independent their entire lives, expressing gratitude may be difficult. Such difficulties also may signal a denial of their condition (Emmons, 2004).

Bruce, a retired educator, came to a hospice facility in San Francisco where I was a bedside volunteer. He had congestive heart failure and was obsessively independent. As he became weaker, Irma, a very considerate staff person, tried to help him. He not only refused all of her efforts but often would yell at her. Allowing anyone to help meant he was dying; something he couldn't accept. Once, after being screamed at and cursed, Irma quietly said, "I know you don't want my help now, but I want you to know, when you can accept it, I'll be here for you."

For two weeks he refused all offers of help, causing himself needless pain. I was alone with him when he had to urinate and realized his urinal was full. With great hesitation he apologetically asked me to empty it. When I returned, he spent the next ten minutes repeatedly thanking me. The gratitude he expressed was totally out of proportion to what I thought I had done. I made the mistake of saying, "It was nothing." In my mind, what I did was routine. To Bruce, asking me to empty a urinal meant the acceptance of dependence and his terminal condition.

### *What to Do*

- When someone offers thanks, accept it without qualification.
- Understand that being grateful can be embarrassing.
- The smallest gesture of kindness to a person who is dying can have enormous consequences.

## Regrets

As people approach death, they often have regrets about things they did and those they wish they had done. Regrets often take the form of goals not achieved, apologies owed, and apologies needed. Professionals are inclined either to minimize these concerns or to switch the conversation to less painful topics. Unless resolved, however, such concerns may be barriers to a more peaceful death for the patient.

## Unmet Goals

Western civilization is goal-driven. We strive to achieve specific things: to amass money, to live comfortably, to become a successful SLP. Our patients also are a product of the society in which they live (Weber, 1946). They are as logs floating down a river. Although each moves differently, all are being carried downstream by the flow of water. Patients whose lives have been goal-directed often focus on things they haven't achieved, regardless of their accomplishments. If they dwell on such things as they approach death, it is significant, even if, in the general scheme of life, it's not.

I cared for a well-known journalist who had written ten books throughout his illustrious life, and hundreds of newspaper columns during World War II. Many people believed he was responsible for changing how war stories were reported. His prostate cancer had metastasized, and approaching death, he fixated on an unfinished magazine article he knew would never be completed. Despite having accomplished more in his life than most other journalists, he could focus only on the incomplete article—one he acknowledged would be a "minor contribution." It can be difficult to console people who view their lives as a series of unfulfilled dreams.

## Apologies:  To Be Given and Received

We all can identify things we're sorry we did, and for which we would like to receive forgiveness. We also have had painful things done to us we vividly remember years after they occurred. As people approach death, wanting to be forgiven and wanting to forgive become important. For those of you who are runners, it's like a burr in your sock that prevents you from feeling good about your run, no matter how fast it was. Not forgiving or receiving forgiveness can prevent people from having a "good death" (Kapleau, 1989).

When I first met Ethel, an 82-year-old woman with pulmonary failure, her dementia was just beginning. During each of my first three weekly visits, she repeated a story of how she, as an elementary school teacher, was ignored by other teachers in her school. As she told and retold the detailed story, reliving the 40-year-old experience changed a beautiful smiling face into one clearly in pain. I spent many hours with her trying to explore how the other teachers' inadequacies may have caused them to do hurtful things. After two months of conversations, she was finally able to forgive their cruelty. Whether they were justified in snubbing her is moot. My concern was to do whatever was necessary to help her death be more peaceful than it would have been while she harbored 40-year-old resentments.

### What to Do

- Let patients express their regrets and acknowledge the importance of such expression to them.
- Help them examine the factors beyond their control that prevented them from achieving goals.
- Try to redirect the focus to things they did achieve without minimizing what they didn't.
- If the patient needs to be forgiven by someone who is still alive, help him or her construct the dialogue to express it. If those people are dead, or not available to receive the apology, ask the patient to imagine you are that person and role-play. Alternatively, have the patient dictate a letter to the person.
- If the patient wants to forgive someone, use the same procedures cited for being forgiven.
- Help the patient understand that often the meanness people perpetrate is a reflection of their own needs, rather suggesting anything negative about the patient.

## Simplification

One of the tenets of most Eastern religions and philosophies is the importance of simplifying life (Hanh, 2000). Although it is a choice for how we live, it becomes a necessity for most people who are dying. Life, for many, is analogous to a complicated musical piece, such as Mahler's *Fifth Symphony* or Billy Strayhorn's *Take the A Train*. In both, it's possible to hear numerous instruments, the melody, the chord changes, the variations, and on and on. But to really understand the piece, it must be reduced to the basic melody. For people who are dying, it's the melody of their lives they strive to hear. It is accomplished through a stripping-away process, wherein most unimportant things are disregarded.

This is true for adults and children, although the stripping-away will be expressed differently in each age group. For example, with children, safety comes from being quietly held by an adult, rather than playing with their familiar toys. Adults give up pretenses and ignore social niceties, and as egos dissolve, role-related behaviors stop. At all ages, verbal communication dwindles. Unfortunately, many people misinterpret this as "withdrawal." The stripping-away process can take many forms. Sometimes it's subtle, as when a person who was on top of current events no longer cares to read a newspaper. Other times it's more blatant, as when a well-known poet decided to give herself a going-away party. She invited friends to her hospice facility, and after everyone told her how she changed their lives, she called each person individually to her side. In a whisper, she said something and then gave each a single sheet of paper on which one of her poems was written. When all of her poems were given away, she turned calmly to everyone and softly said, "Now, I'm ready to die."

Few simplification processes are as dramatic as that one. But you will see it happen with everyone. It's almost as if the person is preparing for a trip to a foreign country and is limited to carrying 50 pounds in baggage. What is this person going to take? This choice, for your patients, will determine how they die. I was with a woman who was actively dying and talked about terrible things in her life. She was agitated and frightened. I reminded her of the intense love she felt for her granddaughter, and helped her to simplify her thoughts by eliminating everything except the image of her granddaughter cuddled next to her in bed.

### What to Do

- Understand that past interests may fade away as the person approaches death.
- Recognize that interests will become basic: Are people listening to me? Do people love me? What do I need for this journey?
- Help patients focus on the most important things that give them peace.

## Techniques for Facilitating Painful Communication

Communication is multi-dimensional. We do it through our thoughts, words, touch, presence, and even silence. If done correctly, it can heal the soul of the person who is dying and give comfort to family and friends.

### Listen

The need to listen can be placed on a long continuum. At one end are people who believe there is little or nothing to be learned from their students. At the other end are people who view everything in life as a source of knowledge. Probably at no time in our experience as communication counselors is it more important to recognize the knowledge inherent (the expertise) in those with whom we counsel.

Most people who are dying, whether an 85-year-old with metastasized cancer or a 6-year-old with cystic fibrosis, are in greater need of someone willing to listen than they are of someone ready to act or solve problems in their behalf (Goldberg, 2005a). It has been noted many times in this book that one of the hardest things for us as professionals to do is listen without judging. It's essential to understand that our patients know more about their needs and condition than we do (Goldberg, 1997). And if we just listen, we may become as knowledgeable as they are.

Many believe that as someone approaches death, the person's need to communicate diminishes. Actually, the reverse is true. Unfortunately, we misperceive a reduction in words as a reduction in need. People who are dying are facing the most profound transition they will ever encounter. Everything about them is changing. Silence in the dying may signal great uncertainty or fear, not the desire to be uncommunicative. Sogyal Rinpoche has said that speaking is for entertainment, but silence is for great wisdom (1994).

Listening is curative, both to the person who is being listened to and the one listening. Most people who are dying desperately want to talk about their lives and their deaths with someone who will silently, nonjudgmentally listen. As a hospice volunteer, I've often listened to people coming to terms with the end of their life: an 86-year-old who reviewed a life of blessings; a teenager whose only regret was the emotional pain he was causing his mother; a child realizing she will never become a ballerina. I've also listened to the last breaths of a woman as I silently held her hand and felt the pain she experienced living on the street her entire adult life. The most profound communication came from a dying infant I held in my arms as her life refused to leave.

Listening is more than not talking. It becomes the ability to be in tune with a person's needs, whether it's breathing in unison or holding the hand of someone struggling with pain that can't be dulled by morphine.

We are uncomfortable with silence; often filling it with word-fluff that does little more than mark time until something of significance can be said. As professionals, we need to resist this temptation.

### What to Do

- When you are with a dying person, sit closely with the chair facing the bed.
- Don't assume that silence means there is no desire to communicate.
- Silence is a form of communication.
- Simplify emotionally difficult concepts.
- Allow your patient to choose the discussion topics.

## Using Healing Communications

People who are dying often have a heightened sense of awareness—they are looking for anything that will help them understand their lives and accept their deaths. Assume everything you say has importance. That doesn't mean you need to fret over every word. Rather, if you understand your role, needless verbiage is naturally reduced. It's also useful to think about words as only one way of communicating. You can "talk" by touch, nonverbal behaviors, playing a soothing instrument such as a Native American flute, and just being present. When I'm with patients, "words" are the least desirable method of developing a bond. If I can convey a feeling through any other means of communication, I do.

I was asked to visit a homeless schizophrenic who was dying of lung cancer at a hospice facility. During my first visit, he didn't say more than 20 words. As I sat next to him, he would occasionally glance at me and then quickly avert his eyes. After nearly an hour of silence, I said, "I have to go now. Thank you for letting me visit with you. Would you like me to come back next week?" I expected him to either remain silent or say "no." Instead, without any hesitation and while looking directly at me, he said, "Yes. I'd like that a lot."

Our second meeting began as the first did. Then, after about 15 minutes of silence, he said, "I'm afraid of dying. Do you know what it's like?" I told him what I had experienced with the deaths of other people. We talked for over half an hour, with him initiating the topics that concerned him. My role was to help him formulate into words those things that previously were too frightening to talk or even think about.

### What to Do

- Don't rush to fill the silence.
- Touch, if the patient feels comfortable with it.
- Listen more, talk less. Think about listening 80% of the time.
- Keep noise to a minimum.

## Witnessing

"Witnessing" is not used here in a religious sense. It simply means acknowledging the person's condition and what they are experiencing. Witnessing a person's terminal illness, nonjudgmentally, can be one of the greatest gifts you can give—not just as a communication counselor but also as a caring person. It requires compassion: the ability to place oneself in another's shoes. It may be difficult to feel compassion for people who brought on their own demise, such as a lifelong smoker, a drug addict, or someone who practiced unsafe sex. Thich Nhat Hanh, a Vietnamese monk, thought it was possible to feel compassion for anyone by visualizing the person as one's mother (Hanh, 1991). After all, how could you deny love to someone who nurtured you when you were helpless? I found the visualization useful when I cared for Bill, a man who was dying of hepatitis.

Every Friday we would drive to Lands End, a scenic place in San Francisco, and watch the Golden Gate Bridge to our right and the Pacific Ocean to our left. As Bill smoked his medical marijuana to stop the nausea from his pain medication, he talked about his life. As much as I wanted to probe, it was important for him to tell someone his life story, without being judged. So I rarely asked questions. And when I did, it was for clarification. Although his lifestyle and some of his values were different from mine, I was there not to judge, but to allow him to communicate. At one of our last outings he told me of events in his life he never shared with anyone. When he finished, he looked more peaceful than he ever had before. He said he felt comfortable telling me because he needed to talk about these life events without being judged.

### What to Do

- Don't impose your needs or understanding of how the world should be.
- Accept your patient's view of how the world is for that person.
- View your patients with compassion, regardless of what they have done with their lives.
- Treat each patient as if he or she were your mother (or another beloved older relative if that works better).
- Stand with the patient as the dying process progresses.
- Figuratively and literally hold the patient's hand.

## The Language of Dying

There was a time, in the Middle Ages, when dying wasn't considered a big deal (Moller, 1996). You knew something irreversible was happening to your body despite ingesting ancient and blessed potions.

You made peace with everyone, tied up loose ends, gave away the furniture, and then just stopped breathing. Now we're afraid to use the "D" word and avoid referring to it, even indirectly, in our hello's and goodbye's.

## Using the "D" Word

In the 1930s there was a notion that labeling a child as a "stutterer" would lead to severe psychological trauma (Van Riper, 1939). Somewhat illogically, it was thought that despite being teased for repeating and blocking, children who stuttered would not perceive themselves as different from other children. We often do the same thing with people who are dying. Family and friends are afraid of using the "D" word, although these people are aware what's happening to them. When patients corner physicians for an answer regarding how long they have to live, even the most brilliant clinicians stumble as if they were on a first date.

I volunteer at George Mark Children's House hospice, located in San Leandro, California. Although we don't initiate conversations about dying with children, parents know that if their child asks us, we won't lie. I remember playing with a 7-year-old boy whose health was rapidly deteriorating. We had gotten close since he had entered the House. As it became harder for him to roll balls to me in a game we had designed, he said, "We won't be able to do this anymore, will we?" I asked him why he thought that and he said, "I think I'm getting closer to dying." I put my arms around him and didn't say anything.

Most adults know they're dying even when you don't use the word. And so do many children. I've seen 6-year-olds realize it. Younger children, who may not have a concept of death, also know something very different is happening—you can see it in their behaviors. There is a misguided notion that pretending someone isn't dying will reduce the trauma. "Ignorance is bliss" works only when everything surrounding the person is conforming to the deception. Yes, the realization that one is dying can be a terrifying experience. Unless the accompanying deterioration is extremely rapid, a person eventually will realize it. The moment of knowing one is going to die is shocking, but for many, it is not as traumatic as reviewing their lives after receiving the news. Difficult deaths

occur when people can't tie up the loose ends or don't have sufficient time to do it.

### What to Do

- Determine the institution's/family's position on talking about death.
- If children ask if they are dying, ask them why they think they are.
- If your patient wants to talk about dying, don't change the subject.
- Don't be afraid to use the words "death" and "dying" if your patient has used them.
- Don't use euphemisms such as "passing on" or "passing away," unless your patient uses them first.
- Mourning isn't confined to friends and relatives of the deceased. People who are dying mourn the losses they have already experienced and the ones they will undergo. Don't be afraid to talk about it.

## Greetings and Goodbyes

When greeting patients, we often use stock lines such as "How are you?" Once, I actually had a patient answer: "I'm dying." So there are better ways of expressing concern, such as "How have you been this week? or "How has your pain been?" Sometimes it's eas-ier to ask about specific behaviors. A hospice nurse I know always starts her visit with "How's it going?"

Leaving poses another linguistic problem. There is a natural tendency to say, "Goodbye, I'll see you next week." But terminally ill patients know there may not be a next week. In some ways, the phrase perpetuates the fiction. A better approach is to express how much the visit meant to you. I often say, "Thanks for allowing me to visit this week. I enjoyed the time we spent together."

### What to Do

- When greeting, focus on specific behaviors, not general health.
- When leaving, express your appreciation for the visit; don't say that you'll see the person the following week.

## Learning from Our Patients

Shared expertise has been a theme of this book. The point has been made that considering ourselves as experts who talk and make suggestion to which others listen and then act on is probably not a good idea. It *really* doesn't work with people who are dying. Don't be afraid of becoming involved in your clients' lives. If you do, you'll receive the greatest lessons on living.

## Getting Involved

We hear the often-touted belief that professional distance is a necessary attribute (Maslach, 1993). We are warned that getting close with someone will lead to a loss of objectivity or, worse, to caring too much. Well-meaning instructors counsel us: "Don't take your cases home with you—that's the quickest way of burning out." I began experiencing the cost of such involvement early in my hospice work, when during my first month, four of the residents whom I became close to died. Fortunately, at the time a presentation was scheduled by a nurse who, for 15 years, had been involved in hospice work. I asked her how she had been able to accept the loss of the thousands she cared for—how was it possible not to get professional burnout. Her answer was illuminating:

> "Love can take many forms. The love I experience for my patients involves feeling I've done everything I could have to make their death as peaceful as possible. I know everyone I care for will die within six months. If I focused on that, I'd go crazy or quit. But when you know you're helping them on a journey, your love is different. So is your sense of loss. Yes, I miss most of the patients I've worked with, but that's minor compared with what I think I gave them."

Caring too much doesn't result in burnout. Actually, I've found the reverse to be true. I've never left a bedside quite the same person I was when I sat down. Instead of feeling drained, I'm invigorated. Compassion is a strange drug. You'll find that the more you give, the more you'll receive. Often, the gifts come in the form of lessons.

### What to Do

- Understand that you're not there to fix anything. All of your terminally ill patients will die, no matter what you do.
- Burnout doesn't come from caring too much. It comes from not realizing that your role is to help the transition between life and death.

## The Lessons

Sogyal Rinpoche (1995) noted that the Buddha said that just as an elephant leaves the biggest footprint in the jungle, so does death when it comes to living. When you are in the presence of someone who will soon die, you probably will have your greatest opportunity for learning how to live. I learned the importance of *forgiveness* from an ex-heroin addict whose family took grim pleasure in the fact that he was dying, because they blamed him for the death of his son. I also learned the power of *compassion*, watching an elderly angry woman dramatically change her life one month before she died in my arms. I learned the need for *friendship* from the founder of a historic collection of gay erotic art, afraid he would die alone. I learned *selflessness* from a teenager suffering from cystic fibrosis, who was more concerned about the distress he was causing his mother than the pain he experienced with each breath. And I learned *living in the present* from a woman who, while holding her infant and knowing he would be dead within a few days, thanked friends and family for a surprise Mother's Day party.

These persons and others provided profound lessons that grabbed me and said, "Listen, this is important." I was able to recognize the offering of such lessons only after I redefined my role from an SLP to a communication counselor. Even though I wasn't functioning in a professional capacity in hospice, I brought my professional orientation with me (Goldberg, 2005b). Throughout my career, I viewed what I did as "fixing" or "helping." I worked with children and *fixed* a language problem. With adults, I *helped* persons with aphasia regain the ability to retrieve words or stutterers how to use fluency-enhancing strategies. How you view what is done in therapy makes a difference in your development as a person.

According to Remen in her book *Kitchen Table Wisdom: Stories That Heal*, when you *fix*, you assume something is broken (Remen, 1997). When you *help*, you see the person as weak. With either perception, there is unequal relationship. It's the one-way street we've gone down our entire professional lives. But when you *serve*, you see the person as intrinsically whole, and create a relationship in which both of you grow. The focus shifts from inequities to abilities; to what each can teach the other. As a hospice volunteer, I don't try to fix or help. I serve, and in the process learn how to live from those who are dying. As communication specialists, you can do the same.

### What to Do

- Regardless of the disease or the severity, view your patients as whole human beings.
- Listen to people who are dying; they have profound insights into living—what to do and what to avoid.
- If possible, be present at the death of your patient. It's the greatest spiritual event you'll ever witness—other than your own death.

## Conclusions

There is a Cherokee saying that "the heart is the first teacher." As threatening as it may be, allow it to open with dying patients. The poet Rilke said that "our deepest fears are like dragons guarding our deepest treasures" (Mitchell, 1989). Your patients hold the keys to your locked doors.

## References

Emmon, R. A. (2004). The psychology of gratitude: An introduction. In R. A. Emmons & M. E. McCullough (Eds.), *The psychology of gratitude* (pp. 3–16). New York: Oxford University Press.

Goldberg, S. A. (1997). *Clinical skills for speech-language pathologists.* San Diego, CA: Singular Publishing Group.

Goldberg, S. 2002). Reinvent yourself: 10 principles of change. *Psychology Today, October,* 38–44.

Goldberg, S. A. (2003). Are we losing our heart? *ASHA Leader, June.*

Goldberg, S. (2005a). A life changed: Lessons learned as a hospice volunteer, *SFSU Magazine, Winter*(5), 1.

Goldberg, S. (2005b). *Ready to learn: How to help your preschooler succeed.* New York: Oxford University Press.

Goldberg, S. (2006). Shedding your fears: Bedside etiquette for dying patients. *Topics in Stroke Rehabilitation, 13*(1), 63–67.

Hanh, T. N. (1991). *Peace is every step.* New York: Bantam Books.

Hanh, T. N. (2000). *The path of emancipation.* Berkeley, CA: Parallax Press.

Kapleau, P. (1989). *The zen of living and dying.* Boston: Shambhala.

Korzybski A. (1958). *Science and sanity.* Lakeville, CT: The International Non-Aristotelian Library.

Krishnamurti, J. (1994) *Commentaries on living.* Madras, India: Quest Books.

Kübler-Ross, E. (1997). *On death and dying.* New York: Scribner.

Maslach, C. (1993). Burnout: A multidimensional perspective. In W. B. Scheaufel, C. Maslach, & T. Marek (Eds.), *Professional burnout: Recent developments in theory and research* (pp. 19–32). New York: CRC Publishers.

Mitchell, S. (Trans.). (1989). *The selected poetry of Maria Rilke.* New York: Vintage Press.

Moller, D. W. (1996). *Confronting death.* New York: Oxford University Press.

Remen, R. (1997). *Kitchen table wisdom: Stories that heal.* New York: Riverhead.

Rinpoche, P. (1994). *The words of my perfect teacher.* Boston: Shambhala.

Rinpoche, S. (1993). *Tibetan wisdom for living and dying.* (Audiotape.) New York: Rigpa Foundation.

Rinpoche, S. (1994). *The Tibetan book of living and dying.* New York: HarperSanFrancisco.

Rinpoche, S. (1995). *Glimpse after glimpse.* New York: HarperSanFrancisco.

Van Riper, C. (1939). *Speech correction: Principles and methods.* New York: Prentice Hall.

Weber, M. (1946). *Essays in sociology.* New York: Oxford University Press.

# INDEX

**F**

**G**

*S*